Diver Medical Technician

Care of the Injured Diver:

Workbook and Exam Review

Commander Ronald L. Ellerman (ret.)

No part of this book may be reproduced, transmitted, or stored in any form or by any means electronic or mechanical, including photocopying, recording, scanning, digitizing, or by any information storage or retrieval system, without the expressed written consent of the author.

Diver Medical Technician – Care of the Injured Diver: Workbook and Exam Review

By Ronald L. Ellerman

© Copyright 2018 by Ronald L. Ellerman. All Rights Reserved

Original photography and illustrations © Copyright 2011-2018 by Ronald L. Ellerman unless otherwise noted. All Rights Reserved

LifeArt illustrations used under license from LifeART / MediClip Images. © Copyright 2011 by Wolters Kluwer Health, Inc. - Lippincott Williams & Wilkins. All Rights Reserved.

Cover Design: Ronald L. Ellerman

Disclaimer

This workbook is intended to be utilized in the teaching of a medical course by qualified and knowledgeable instructors in the procedures and treatments contained herein. It is not intended to be utilized as a self-study or self-taught guide.

The procedures and protocols in this workbook are based on the most current recommendations and practices of responsible medical sources. Hyperbaric Training Associates, the author, and the publisher, however, make no guarantee as to, and assume no responsibility for, the correctness, sufficiency, or completeness of such information or recommendations. Other or additional safety and medical measures may be required under particular circumstances. The medical field is extremely dynamic with regards to new procedures and equipment. Readers are encouraged and advised to check the most current information provided, on procedures featured, and by the manufacturer of each product featured. To the fullest extend of the law, neither Hyperbaric Training Associates, the author, nor the publisher assumes any liability for any injury and/or damage to persons or property arising out of or related to any use of the material contained in this textbook.

This workbook is intended solely as a guide to the appropriate measures and procedures to be utilized and employed when rendering emergency care to the sick and injured. It is not intended as a statement of the standard of care required in any particular situation or circumstance, due to the fact that circumstances and patient conditions may vary widely from one emergency to another. Nor is it intended that this workbook shall, in any way, advise emergency medical personnel concerning legal authority to perform the activities and procedures discussed herein. Such determination shall be made locally and with the aid of legal council only.

Users of this workbook are further warned that the use of any technique, procedure, treatment, drug, or other substance must be authorized by their medical control and direction through standing orders, protocols, or online consultation and direction and must also, where appropriate, be in accordance with local, state, federal, and international laws and regulations.

Gender Statement

The English language has historically given preference to the male gender. In many cases, the pronouns, he and his, are commonly used to describe both genders. Since the male pronouns still dominate our speech and language, they have been used throughout this workbook to portray both male and female diver medics and patients for brevity. The author realizes and acknowledges that female divers and diver medics play an important and indispensable role in this industry and this usage in no way diminishes their importance.

About the Author

Ronald Ellerman, BS, AAS, retired from the Fire Service as a Shift Commander with over 32 years' experience. Commander Ellerman, along with his normal firefighting duties, acted as the commanding chief officer for the Emergency Medical Service and Special Operations divisions of the fire department. He was involved in every facet of EMS and Special Operations from training, protocol and operational development, equipment specification, and purchasing. He has been a licensed Emergency Medical Technician Instructor Coordinator since the mid-1980s and a Diver Medical Technician instructor for over 15 years, developing and conducting a variety of medical training programs including Emergency Medical Technician, Advanced Prehospital Trauma Life Support, Remote Duty Medic, Tactical Emergency Medical Technician, and Diver Medical Technician.

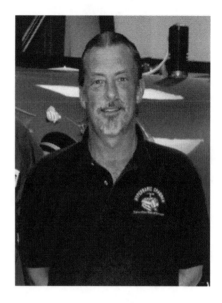

CMDR. Ronald L. Ellerman

His diving career began with the fire service in the mid-1970s as a public safety and inland commercial diver. Commander Ellerman has been involved in various aspects of diving and diver training, including advanced training in response to diver emergencies. Students he has trained over the years in his DMT program include military, special operations, commercial off-shore, saturation, and recreational divers, along with emergency medical personnel who respond to diver emergencies. He currently works with, and supports, one of the worlds' busiest hyperbaric chambers for diving injuries located in Central America and has done so for the past 22 years. This work has allowed him to be involved in the treatment of hundreds, upon hundreds, of Miskito Indian lobster divers who have suffered severe Type II DCS injuries along with injured recreational divers.

Currently, Commander Ellerman and Cornerstone Medical Services hold dual accreditation from both the National Board of Diving and Hyperbaric Medical Technology and the International Marine Contractors Association as a Diver Medic training facility and instructor.

Using This Workbook

This workbook has been written as a companion text for 'Diver Medical Technician – Care of the Injured Diver'. The content of this workbook follows the main text of that book and provides numerous questions and activities that can be easily completed if the student has read and studied the accompanying text.

Instructors have the option to use the various review sections as teaching assignments for each portion of the Diver Medic classes. Meaning, Section One of the workbook would be completed either prior to, or immediately following the Section One lesson.

Students can use this workbook as a study guide and review for their certification examination. The National Board of Diving and Hyperbaric Technology (NBDHMT) now require the Diver Medic candidate to sit for a NBDHMT administered certification examination. This workbook should cover all of the subject areas that the NBDHMT examination covers.

The International Marine Contractors Association (IMCA) allows the training facilities and faculty to administer their own certification examinations that have been approved by IMCA. Again, this workbook covers the all of the subject areas that a candidate would find on an IMCA certification examination.

The Examinations

As stated above, IMCA examinations are administered through the IMCA approved training centers. The NBDHMT requires the Diver Medic candidate to sit for a NBDHMT administered certification examination.

Both agencies utilize multiple-choice formats with IMCA also utilizing oral examination of various subject areas.

The following pages show the breakdown that was provided to DMT instructors by the NBDHMT as to the contents and weight for each subject that will be contained in the NBDHMT certification examination. As of August 2018, this breakdown was current and being used in the NBDHMT testing process.

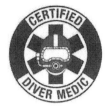 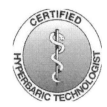 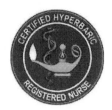 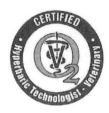

National Board of Diving & Hyperbaric Medical Technology

NBDHMT DMT Certification Examination Guidelines

DMT certification is based upon a series of mandatory pre-requisites. They include:

1. Completion of a NBDHMT approved DMT training course
2. Completion of formal medical first responder training
3. Medically determination of fitness to work in pressurized environments

Once all of the above have been satisfactory undertaken the DMT can apply to take the DMT certification examination.

The DMT examination test bank comprised of questions from seven categories. All questions are multiple-choice and have only one correct answer. No questions are designed to trick the examinee. Listed below are the seven categories, topics covered within each category, the percentage of questions from the entire examination that are derived from each category, and how many questions each respective percentage represents. Numerous variations of the DMT examination question bank are in use at any given time. A scientific calculator may be used.

Category 1: Physics and Physiology

Defining pressure (absolute, gauge, barometric); measuring pressure (standard/imperial, metric); converting pressure (absolute to gauge- gauge to absolute in mmHg, psig, psia, fsw, msw, ATA); converting between degrees Fahrenheit and degrees Celsius; gas law definitions and computations (Boyle's, Dalton's, Henry's and Charles's/Guy-Lussac's); computing oxygen percent and oxygen/nitrogen partial pressures involving various depths and various breathing mixtures; factors influencing inert gas uptake and elimination; USN definitions of treatment and emergency gases.

Nine Category 1 questions are selected from the examination question bank. They represent 7.5% of the total questions in each individual examination.

Category 2: Decompression Sickness & Cerebral Arterial Gas Embolism

Basic pathophysiology of decompression illness; surface orientated and saturation diving induced cases; symptom presentation; differential diagnosis Type 1 vs. Type 2 *DCS*, DCS-CAGE, inner ear DCS- inner ear barotrauma; risk factors;

Eighteen Category 2 questions are selected from the examination question bank. They represent 15% of the total questions in each individual examination.

Category 3: Patient Assessment

Shock; Glasgow Coma Scale; extremity injuries; anticipated physical and/or neurological findings in DCS, CAGE, ear and other barotraumas, pneumothorax, tension pneumothorax, subcutaneous emphysema; differential diagnosis; tuning fork hearing acuity testing; otoscopic findings in barotrauma and infection; omitted decompression.

Thirty Category 3 questions are selected from the examination question bank. They represent 25% of the total questions in each individual examination.

Category 4: Recompression Treatment & Decompression Procedures

US Navy treatment of surface orientated and saturation diving-induced DCS; US Navy treatment procedures for CAGE; incomplete relief of DCS during treatment and upon surfacing; omitted decompression.

Twenty-seven Category 4 questions are selected from the examination question bank. They represent 22.5%-of the total questions in each individual examination.

Category 5: Invasive Procedures

Emergent/field management of pneumothorax; routes-of medication administration; nasogastric tubes; wound closure; sterile technique; airway control; Foley catheters; intravenous fluid administration and drip rate calculations; endotracheal tubes; dosing conversions, mg to ml; potential compression complications for ampoules, vials and fluid infusion bottles; Heimlich valves.

Twelve Category 5 questions are selected from the examination question bank. They represent 10% of the total questions in each individual examination.

Category 6: Other Diving Related Injuries, Side Effects & Complications

Central nervous system oxygen toxicity; pulmonary oxygen toxicity; barotraumas; marine envenomation, stings and bites; nitrogen narcosis; hypothermia.

Eighteen Category 6 questions are selected from the examination question bank. They represent 15% of the total questions in each individual examination.

Category 7: Chamber, Equipment and Operational Safety

Diagnostic equipment precautions under pressure; chamber ventilation; chamber fire precautions; atmospheric sampling; tender/medic decompression safety.

Six Category 7 questions are selected from the examination question bank. They represent 5% of the total questions in each individual examination.

Diver Medical Technician

Care of the Injured Diver: Workbook and Exam Review

Commander Ronald L. Ellerman (ret.)

Contents

1. *History of Diving and Hyperbarics* 1
2. *Roles and Responsibilities of the Diver Medic* 5
3. *Diving Physics* 7
4. *Anatomy and Physiology Review* 13
5. *Patient Assessment* 21
6. *Tables – Decompression and Recompression* 27
7. *Hyperbaric Chambers* 31
8. *Pressure Injuries / Illness* 35
9. *Environmental and Marine Injuries* 41
10. *Airway and Breathing* 45
11. *Vascular Access and Medication Administration* 51
12. *Soft Tissue Injury* 59
13. *Musculoskeletal Injury* 65
14. *Cardiac Emergencies* 69
17. *Live Bait* 75

Appendix 79

Section Answer Keys 137

1 History of Diving and Hyperbarics

Mix and Match

Match the terms in the first column with the definitions in the second column.

Column 1

1. _____ Breath hold diver
2. _____ Greek divers
3. _____ Scyllias
4. _____ Food, treasure, salvage, war
5. _____ Ama pearl divers
6. _____ Weighted chamber with open bottom
7. _____ John Smeaton
8. _____ Wet Bell
9. _____ SDC
10. _____ HRC
11. _____ Augustus Siebe
12. _____ Henry Fleuss
13. _____ Jacques Cousteau, Emile Gagnon
14. _____ Technical diver
15. _____ Superlite 17

Column 2

a. Female Asian breathhold divers
b. Reason for early man exploring the sea
c. Diver NOT using diving apparatus to explore the sea
d. Early diving bell
e. Early Greek military diver
f. Early divers who gathered sponges
g. Original, modern commercial helmet invented by Kirby-Morgan
h. Hyperbaric Rescue Chamber
i. Father of modern diving
j. Diver making several gas switches during a dive
k. Inventors of modern SCUBA equipment
l. Submersible Diving Chamber
m. Inventor of the first truly functional diving bell
n. Inventor of the first functional rebreather
o. Bubble topped diving bell

Section 1 – History of Diving and Hyperbarics

Review Questions – Multiple Choice

1. In 1919, an American scientist, working for the U.S. Mines Bureau, suggested that helium could be substituted for nitrogen in diving gas mixes.

    a. Dr. Edgar End
    b. Arne Zetterstrom
    c. Dick Rutkowski
    d. Elihu Thompson

2. In 1935, Dr. A. Behnke discovered that nitrogen was the cause of which diving problem?

    a. Rapid cooling
    b. Helium shakes
    c. Narcosis
    d. Joint pain

3. In 1939, what type of diving gas mix was finally utilized to assist in the rescue of crew members from the sunken submarine, USS Squalus?

    a. Air mix
    b. Hydrogen / Oxygen mix
    c. Trimix
    d. Helium / Oxygen mix

4. In 1937, this team proved to the US Navy and British Royal Navy, that helium diving was viable by setting a world record during a dive off the coast of Milwaukee, Wisconsin.

    a. Dr. Edgar End / Max Gene Nohl
    b. Dr. A. Behnke / Emile Gagnon
    c. Dr. Ita Boerema / Jack Browne
    d. Dr. Hall / Darrell Oats

5. Hydrogen gas was utilized by this Swedish engineer to produce a diving mix that could reach depths up to 1000 fsw (303 meters) in the 1940's.

    a. Peter Edel
    b. Arne Zetterstrom
    c. George Bond
    d. Sir Robert Boyle

6. The first reported use of "pressure therapy" was in what year and by whom?

    a. Dr. Orville Cunningham / 1618
    b. Dr. Edgar End / 1935
    c. Dr. Henshaw / 1662
    d. Dr. Ite Boerema / 1955

7. In 1938, Dr. Edgar End, Max Nohl, and Jack Browne entered a hyperbaric chamber in the basement of Milwaukee County Emergency Hospital and conducted the first, intentional _____ dive.

    a. Saturation
    b. Heliox
    c. Trimix
    d. Decompression

8. The first commercial diving saturation dive was conducted in what year?

    a. 1938
    b. 1945
    c. 1965
    d. 1862

Section 1 – History of Diving and Hyperbarics

9. Dr. Orville Cunningham is most famous for what structure?

   a. Steel Ball Hospital
   b. Multi-Lock hyperbaric chamber
   c. Mono-place Hyperbaric chamber
   d. Surgical chamber suite

10. Dr. Cunningham is also famous for an incident, which occurred in 1923 and was the first documented _____ in a hyperbaric chamber.

    a. Fire
    b. Structural failure
    c. Over pressurization
    d. Tender bailout

11. What Italian diver and inventor constructed the first decompression chamber in 1916?

    a. Sophia Loren
    b. Heinrich Dräger
    c. Alberto Gianni
    d. Paul Bert

12. Early work in decompression was conducted on which individuals?

    a. Commercial divers
    b. Saturation divers
    c. Caisson workers
    d. Astronauts

13. Who developed the first workable rebreather in 1878?

    a. Edgar End
    b. Henry Fleuss
    c. Jacques Cousteau
    d. Max Nohl

14. In 1945, _____ _____ set a world depth record in a wet pot in the basement of _____.

    a. Benoit Rouquayrol / Comex
    b. Bill Johnson / Schrader & Sons
    c. Max Nohl / Gimbel's
    d. Jack Browne / DESCO

15. Arne Zetterstrom used hydrogen as a replacement for hard to acquire helium gas. He was limited to using only _____ % of oxygen due to the explosive nature of the mix.

    a. 4   b. 6   c. 8   d. 2

16. The first documented, intentional saturation dive was conducted where?

    a. Panama City, Florida
    b. Amsterdam, Holland
    c. Duke University
    d. Milwaukee, Wisconsin

17. DESCO, and other companies, was producing the _____ _____ _____ during the war and DESCO continues to produce this helmet in its Milwaukee plant.

    a. US Navy Mark V Mod 1
    b. Air hat
    c. Rat Hat
    d. Superlite 17

Section 1 – History of Diving and Hyperbarics

Find the Terms and Names

```
H Y T R E S S J A C K B R O W N E T Y R
O T F L E U S S T K Y K F T N M D E R P
M R D E G B Y P S I E B E P M W G T S O
E O I J O M Q U M Y R Y D W N K A H Q Q
R J R G S E L E E B D D E S C O R E U D
M A R G A R I T A I S L A N D P E D A A
R N F B Y S F E T L V M N W D O N H L D
W W Y H T I T C O M E X E W Y L D S U G
D A M A A B M E G L I S H M E H W A S H
F R I L D L S J S U P E R L I T E T Q K
G S O L W E T B E L L T Q S V H R U R L
H T J Y H B E L L Z E T T E R S T R O M
K L I N G E R T A A T D T A U S Y A Y I
E M R Y K H T T F S H A W L I G J T S L
Y R M A X N O H L S B L U A M J L I R W
H T O N E K I P T V R S P B E Y W O J A
U Y M E D E L N O E I C C A Q U T N K U
J I S M Y D A S W M D U N D E R S E A K
F R E N C H Y E G U G B A R T O B I Y E
S E N O W C O U S T E A U T I W U D L E
```

Jack Browne	Homer	Fleuss
Trojan War	Siebe	Edgar End
Squalus	Submersible	Behnke
HPNS	Klingert	French
Cousteau	Undersea	Saturation
Milwaukee	Superlite	English
Comex	Shaw	Lethbridge
SCUBA	Edel	Momsen
DESCO	Margarita Island	Hally
Wetbell	Zetterstrom	Sealab
Ama	French	Max Nohl

2 Roles and Responsibilities of the Diver Medic

Review Questions - Multiple Choice

1. During an incident, you as a diver medic may be interacting with a Diving Medical Officer (DMO). Acting as the control physician's eyes, ears, and hands.

    a. True
    b. False

2. As a DIVER, the diver medic should do what to insure safe diving practices?

    a. Lead by example
    b. Ignore diving profiles
    c. Maintain other divers equipment
    d. Never voice safety concerns

3. As a MEDIC, the diver medic will be required to act within their "Scope of Practice" as determined by the DMO or company protocols.

    a. True
    b. False

4. Documentation of any patient care provided by the diver medic is required.

    a. True
    b. False

5. In the US, patient information and confidentiality is covered by the what?

    a. Obama Care
    b. Jones Act
    c. HIPPA
    d. Ryan-White Act

6. A diver medic may be called upon to perform routine healthcare procedures while on the job.

    a. True
    b. False

7. Which of the following is NOT a basic vital sign?

    a. Full blood analysis
    b. Blood pressure readings
    c. Pupillary responses
    d. Respiratory rate

8. Initial patient history taking includes, for divers, all of the following except?

    a. Diving history
    b. Medications
    c. Recent medical history
    d. Certification level

9. A diver medic should liaison with other healthcare professional in their response area.

    a. True
    b. False

3 Diving Physics

Matching

Match the terms in the first column with the definitions in the second column.

1. _____ Atmospheric Pressure

2. _____ Atmospheres Absolute

3. _____ Hydrostatic Pressure

4. _____ Pressure

5. _____ Gauge Pressure

6. _____ Ambient Pressure

7. _____ Partial Pressure

8. _____ Boyle's Law

9. _____ Dalton's Law

10. _____ Pascal's Principle

11. _____ Archimedes' Principle

12. _____ Henry's Law

13. _____ Charles Law

14. _____ Gay-Lussac's Law

15. _____ Ideal (General) Gas Law

a. Sum of the gas parts is equal to the total pressure

b. Force acting on all objects

c. Father of the pressure / volume relationship

d. Father of the partial pressure law

e. Hydrostatic plus atmospheric pressures

f. 14.7 psi (760 mmHg) at sea level

g. Atmospheric pressure adjusted gauge reading

h. Surrounding pressure of an object

i. Temperature increase causes volume increase

j. Temperature increase causes pressure increase

k. Defines the interrelationship of all gas components; pressure, volume, temperature.

l. Hydraulic principles is defined by this law

m. Buoyancy and fluid displacement principle

n. Weight of water or fluid on a diver

o. Gas law which explains saturation of inert gas

Section 3 – Diving Physics

Find the Terms

Q	D	T	A	A	B	S	O	L	U	T	E	A	H	E
U	O	D	R	T	B	O	Y	L	E	U	A	L	E	T
L	X	W	A	M	S	T	G	E	N	E	R	A	L	R
H	Y	D	R	O	S	T	A	T	I	C	E	I	Y	I
E	G	R	G	S	I	S	U	Q	H	H	U	M	I	M
N	E	W	O	P	F	H	G	G	F	A	I	H	M	I
R	N	W	N	H	E	E	E	A	G	R	M	N	K	X
Y	S	A	Y	E	D	L	K	Y	E	L	E	M	H	H
F	E	P	A	R	T	I	A	L	L	E	D	E	M	Y
U	H	A	M	I	Q	O	H	U	J	S	E	T	G	D
P	R	S	B	C	E	X	L	S	B	R	S	H	U	R
T	T	C	I	D	E	A	L	S	X	D	H	A	L	O
D	S	A	E	U	H	R	H	A	R	G	O	N	S	G
A	D	L	N	J	Y	F	W	C	A	T	F	E	A	E
D	A	L	T	O	N	B	N	I	T	R	O	G	E	N

Absolute	Hydrogen
Atmosphere	Dalton
Heliox	Henry
Hydrostatic	Oxygen
Helium	Gay Lussac
General	Methane
Boyle	Ideal
Charles	Partial
Archimedes	Gauge
Argon	Ambient
Nitrogen	Pascal

Review Questions – Multiple Choice

1. Gauge pressure is an adjusted reading which, at sea level, should read as what pressure?

    a. Zero   b. 14.7 psi   c. 760 mmHg   d. 33 fsw

2. Ambient pressure is the surrounding atmospheric or hydrostatic pressure exerted on a body.

    a. True   b. False

3. Ambient pressure _____ as a diver ascends from depth.

    a. Increases   b. Decreases

    c. Remains constant   d. None of the above

Section 3 – Diving Physics

4. Hydrostatic pressure is defined as the cumulative weight of a fluid on a diver and results in pressure increases of _____ per 33 fsw (10 meters) of descent.

   a. 33 psi / 380 mmHg
   b. 760 mmHg / 1.0 psi
   c. 14.7 psi / 760 mmHg
   d. 0.21 psi / 15 mmHg

5. Atmospheres absolute (ATA) is the combination of hydrostatic pressure and atmospheric pressure.

   a. True
   b. False

6. Atmospheric pressure is considered 14.7 psi (760 mmHg) at sea level. This is also stated as _____ atmosphere.

   a. 1 ATA
   b. 2 ATA
   c. 3 ATA
   d. 4 ATA

7. A diver at 33 fsw (760 mmHg) is under how many ATA(s) of pressure?

   a. 1 ATA
   b. 2 ATA
   c. 3 ATA
   d. 4 ATA

8. A diver at 99 fsw is under how much pressure absolute?

   a. 14.7 psi / 760 mmHg
   b. 44.1 psi / 2280 mmHg
   c. 58.8 psi / 3040 mmHg
   d. 73.5 psi / 3800 mmHg

9. Calculate the ATA for a saturation diver stored at 660 fsw / 200 meters.

   a. 20 ATA   b. 21 ATA   c. 22 ATA   d. 19 ATA

10. Objects underwater appear to be _____ and _____ than on land.

    a. Closer and larger
    b. Smaller and closer
    c. Further away and larger
    d. Same size as on land

11. The increased density of water compared to air causes _____ of the light rays.

    a. Conduction
    b. Transmission
    c. Radiation
    d. Refraction

12. Sound travels faster or slower underwater?

    a. Faster
    b. Slower

13. It is easy to determine where a sound is coming from underwater.

    a. True
    b. False

14. Water has a thermal conductivity about 25 times that of air.

    a. True
    b. False

Section 3 – Diving Physics

15. Helium as a gas is _____ than nitrogen.

    a. Less dense				b. More dense

    c. Same density				d. None of the above

16. Hydrogen as a gas is _____ than helium.

    a. Less dense				b. More dense

    c. Same density				c. None of the above

17. Hydrogen gas has the same narcotic effect as nitrogen under high partial pressures.

    a. True			b. False

18. Hydrogen is highly explosive when mixed with more than _____ percent oxygen.

    a. 4%			b. 75%

    c. 21%			d. 100%

19. The 'Paul Bert' effect deals with central nervous system toxicity of which gas in high concentration?

    a. Nitrogen			b. Helium

    c. Oxygen			d. Hydrogen

20. High Pressure Nervous Syndrome (HPNS) is caused by helium

    a. True			b. False

21. "Trimix" is a combination of which diving gases?

    a. Oxygen, helium, and nitrogen		b. Oxygen, hydrogen, and helium

    c. Carbon dioxide, air, and helium		d. Oxygen, argon, and helium

22. Convert 75 degrees Fahrenheit to degrees Celsius.

    a. 24		b. 28		c. 30		d. 20

23. Covert 70 degrees Fahrenheit to degrees Celsius.

    a. 24		b. 28		c. 30		d. 21

24. Convert 28 degrees Celsius to degrees Fahrenheit.

    a. 82		b. 90		c. 97		d. 52

25. Convert 15 degrees Celsius to degrees Fahrenheit.

    a. 59		b. 72		c. 68		d. 32

Section 3 – Diving Physics

Using the formula provided, find the gas consumption in standard cubic feet for the divers.

Breathing Gas Formula: SCF required = Number of Divers (P) x ATA x Minutes (M) X Respiratory Minute Volume (RMV).   SCF=P x ATA x M x RMV

Patient at Rest = 0.5 SCF/Minute at surface

Light Work = 0.5 SCF/Minute at surface

Moderate Work = 1.0 SCF/Minute at surface

Heavy Work = 1.5 SCF/Minute at surface

1. Find the SCF for a diver doing heavy work at 99 fsw (30 meters) for 15 minutes.

    a. 22.5 SCF   b. 90.0 SCF

    c. 34.0 SCF   d. 14.7 SCF

2. Your patient is resting during a USNTT5 at 60 fsw. Calculate the oxygen needs for the 60 fsw portion of this treatment. (Hint: First find the Minutes at 60 fsw in the USN TT5 profile.)

    a. 60.2 SCF   b. 22.5 SCF

    c. 14.7 SCF   d. 760 SCF

3. A patient is resting during a USN TT6A Modified using 50/50 heliox. The patient will spend 29 minutes at 165 fsw (50 meters). Calculate the required gas for this portion of the treatment.

    a. 60.2 SCF   b. 87 SCF

    c. 33 SCF   d. 14.7 SCF

4 Anatomy and Physiology Review

Fill In the Blanks

Label the appropriate anatomical structure using the terms to the left.

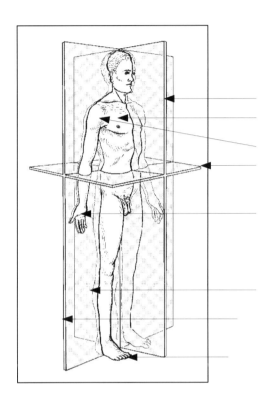

a. Sagittal Plane

b. Midaxillary Plane

c. Midline Plane

d. Dorsal Plane

e. Ventral Plane

f. Plantar

g. Palmar

Label Directional Views

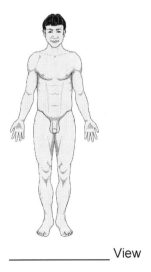
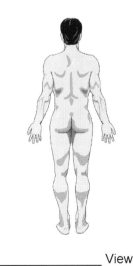
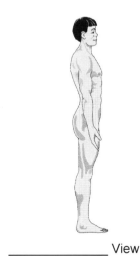

_____ View   _____ View   _____ View

Section 4 – Anatomy and Physiology Review

Label the anatomic parts of the skeleton using the Table to the left.

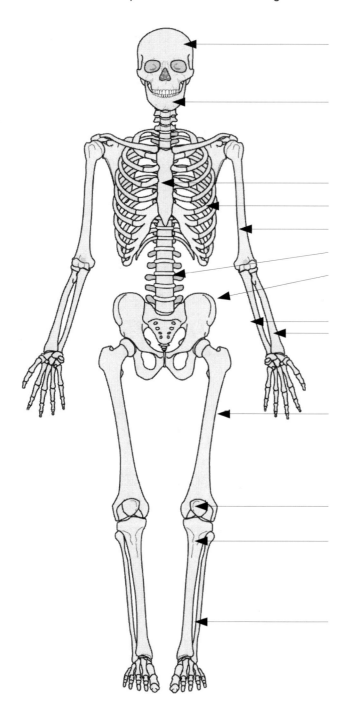

a. Cranium

b. Femur

c. Spinal Column

d. Pelvis

e. Tibia

f. Ulna

g. Rib Cage

h. Patella

i. Fibula

j. Humerus

k. Radius

l. Jaw

m. Sternum

Section 4 – Anatomy and Physiology Review

Label the anatomic parts of the Heart using the Table to the left.

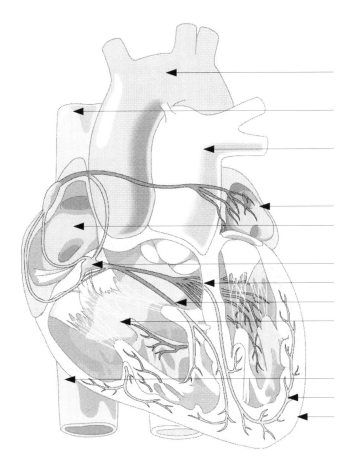

a. Left ventricle

b. Right Ventricle

c. Left Atrium

d. Right Atrium

e. Inferior vena cava

f. Superior vena cava

g. Right bundle branch

h. Left bundle branch

i. Bundle of His

j. Purkinje network

k. Aorta

l. Pulmonary artery

Cardiac Vascular Review Questions – Multiple Choice

1. _____ carry blood to the heart, and _____ carry blood away from the heart.

   a. Capillaries, arteries   b. Capillaries, veins

   c. Veins, arteries   d. Arteries, veins

2. The heart consists of _____ pumping chambers.

   a. 1   b. 2   c. 3   d. 4

3. Plasma is what part of the blood?

   a. Clotting factor   b. Red blood cells

   c. White blood cells   d. Transportation fluid for other blood components

4. Which cells carry oxygen to the cells and remove carbon dioxide?

   a. Platelets   b. Red blood cells

   c. White blood cells   d. Arteries

Section 4 – Anatomy and Physiology Review

5. The primary electrical pacemaker in the right atrium is known as the _____.

    a. Bundle of His   b. AV node

    c. Sinoatrial node   d. Purkinje network

6. The 'QRS' wave of an ECG represents what cardiac function?

    a. Repolarization of the atria   b. Depolarization of the atria

    c. Repolarization of the ventricles   d. Depolarization of the ventricles

7. The 'P' wave of an ECG represents what cardiac function?

    a. Repolarization of the atria   b. Depolarization of the atria

    c. Repolarization of the ventricles   d. Depolarization of the ventricles

8. Veins are blood vessels which contain valves and carries normally lower pressures of blood.

    a. True   b. False

9. Arteries always carry oxygenated blood away from the heart.

    a. True   b. False

10. The heart muscle can tolerate long interruptions of blood supply.

    a. True   b. False

11. A tough, fibrous membrane surrounds the heart. Name this membrane.

    a. Epicardium   b. Endocardium

    c. Visceral pericardium   d. Pericardial sac

12. The capillary beds provide access by the bloodstream, to all body cells.

    a. True   b. False

13. The only veins which carry oxygenated blood are the _____.

    a. Pulmonary veins   b. Inferior vena cava

    c. Superior vena cava   d. Aorta

14. The aorta receives its blood supply from the _____.

    a. Right ventricle   b. Left ventricle

    c. Left atrium   d. Right atrium

15. The heart muscle receives its blood via the coronary arteries.

    a. True   b. False

Section 4 – Anatomy and Physiology Review

Respiratory System Review

Label the anatomic parts of the Upper & Lower Airways using the Table to the left.

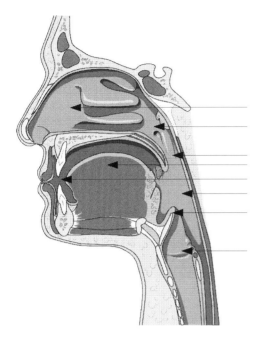

a. Pharynx

b. Nasopharynx

c. Epiglottis

d. Tongue

e. Mouth

f. Larynx

g. Nasal air passage

h. Oropharynx

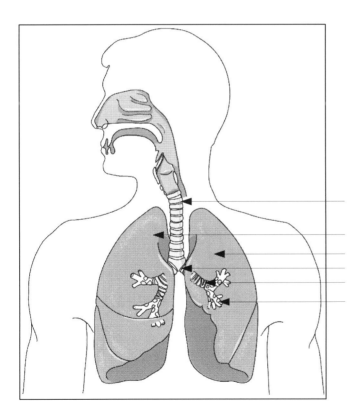

a. Bronchioles

b. Trachea

c. Carina

d. Left Lung

e. Right Lung

f. Mainstream Bronchus

Section 4 – Anatomy and Physiology Review

Respiratory Review Questions – Multiple Choice

1. What muscles are responsible for the ventilation process?

    a. Interstitial, parietal
    b. Inhalation, exhalation
    c. Diaphragm, intercostal
    d. Thoracic, sternal

2. The process of moving air into and out of the lungs is known as _____

    a. Cellular ventilation
    b. Cellular perfusion
    c. Ventilation
    d. Respiration

3. The process which takes place in the alveoli is known as _____

    a. Respiration
    b. Ventilation
    c. Cellular perfusion
    d. Choking

4. The lungs are comprised of how many lobes?

    a. 2
    b. 3
    c. 4
    d. 5

5. The alveoli are surrounded by what type of blood vessels?

    a. Arteries
    b. Veins
    c. Capillaries
    d. Blood cells

6. The exchange of gases takes place in the _____.

    a. Trachea
    b. Larynx
    c. Alveoli
    d. Carina

7. The mainstream bronchi begin and end where?

    a. Larynx, thorax
    b. Carina, alveoli
    c. Oropharynx, nasopharynx
    d. Epiglottis, larynx

8. The lungs are lined with a slippery membrane known as the _____.

    a. Visceral pleura
    b. Parietal pleura
    c. Pericardial sac
    d. Surfactant

9. The thoracic cavity is lined with a slippery membrane known as the _____.

    a. Visceral pleura
    b. Parietal pleura
    c. Pericardial sac
    d. Surfactant

Section 4 – Anatomy and Physiology Review

Nervous System Review

Label the anatomic parts of the Brain using the Table to the left.

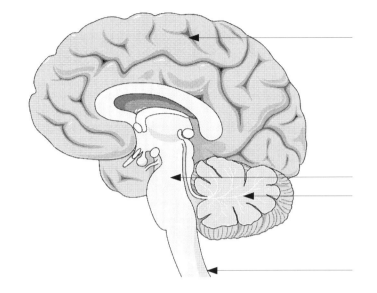

a. Brain stem

b. Spinal cord

c. Cerebellum

d. Cerebrum

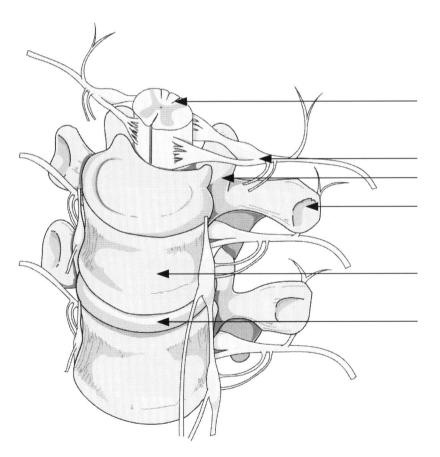

a. Vertebrae body

b. Cartilaginous disk

c. Spinous process

d. Transverse process

e. Nerve

f. Spinal cord

Section 4 – Anatomy and Physiology Review

Find the Terms

```
P E T Y L E F T H M R Y K W C T A V P U
O T P S A D D U C T I O N M I E L B O W
N H O A T R I U M G G R T Y R N W N A R
S E S E E F T M H T H E F O C V A D U I
A N T E R I O R A F T T R C U E T N T S
B W E Q A R T R A C H E A A L N L C O T
D E R U L R B N R E S P I R A T I O N S
U B I L A T E R A L R I K D T R G L O U
C E O L O D E W V W K G K I I I A L M B
T P R O X I M A L L N L M U O C M A I C
I S D R I S R L T Y E O C M N L E G C U
O C M O M T C Y X A E T Z E W E N E J T
N R A P E A H E A R T T Y L N T T N L A
A I R H T L E O I T O I Q A U H G N T N
B C R A R R T L Y E U S S R I O R P P E
O O O R Y K M I S R W R P Y T R C A B O
N I W Y F E M U R Y S P I N E A T I P U
E D E N A S O P H A R Y N X T C H N R S
A P T X R O M B E R G T A T R I C E P L
S Y N A P S E W G K R I L H A C B E T S
```

Posterior	Epiglottis	Marrow
Anterior	Respiration	Ligament
Adduction	Circulation	Knee
Abduction	Heart	Spinal
Proximal	Artery	Thoracic
Distal	Atrium	Elbow
Lateral	Myocardium	Wrist
Bilateral	Ventricle	Collagen
Left	Pons	Subcutaneous
Right	Larynx	PPE
Nasopharynx	Spine	AVPU
Cricoid	Autonomic	Oximetry
Oropharynx	Synapse	Romberg
Trachea	Bone	Pain
Alveoli	Femur	Tricep

5 Patient Assessment
Matching

Match the terms in the first column with the definitions in the second column

1. _____ BSI
2. _____ PPE
3. _____ Scene safety
4. _____ NOI
5. _____ MOI
6. _____ General impression
7. _____ Responsiveness
8. _____ Chief complaint
9. _____ Triage
10. _____ Palpate
11. _____ Auscultate
12. _____ Orientation

a. Equipment wore to prevent BSI exposure.
b. Reason for the call for help.
c. Systematic sorting of patients for treatment
d. Listening
e. Feeling
f. Mental status
g. Nature of Illness
h. Process of securing a scene.
i. Process of avoiding exposure to body fluids.
j. Mechanism of Injury
k. Patient response to external stimulus
l. Overall initial appearance of the patient.

Patient Assessment Review Questions – Multiple Choice

1. Scene safety concerns include all of the following except:

    a. Determining NOI/MOI   b. Need for additional resources

    c. BSI / PPE precaution   d. Auscultation of breath sounds

2. With regards to scene safety, who is the most important person at the scene?

    a. Yourself   b. Your partner   c. The life support technician   d. The patient

3. The fact that your patient acknowledges your presence when you arrive is important?

    a. True   b. False

4. For the patient in question 3, what does this response mean to the diver medic?

    a. Orientation   b. Confusion

    c. Unconsciousness   d. Doubt

Section 5 – Patient Assessment

5. In assessment of mental status, what does the A stand for in AVPU?

    a. Altered	b. Alert

    c. Annoyed	d. Anxious

6. In assessment of mental status, what does the P stand for in AVPU?

    a. Patient	b. Perplexed

    c. Pain	d. Provocation

7. The best indicator of brain function is the patient's what?

    a. Skin color	b. Mental status

    c. Combativeness	d. Pulse rate

8. Which of the following is a symptom?

    a. Cyanosis	b. Headache

    c. Tachycardia	d. Hypertension

9. When you inspect a patient's pupils with a penlight, the pupils should normally react to the light by:

    a. Constricting	b. Enlarging

    c. Dilating	d. Blinking

10. When you shine a light into one pupil, the normal reaction of the other pupil should be to:

    a. Dilate	b. Not react

    c. Become larger	d. Become smaller

11. What maneuver should be used to open the airway of an unresponsive patient with suspected trauma?

    a. Tongue-Jaw lift	b. Jaw-Thrust maneuver

    c. Head Tilt-Chin lift	d. Head Tilt-Neck lift

12. If a patient develops difficulty breathing after your primary assessment, you should immediately:

    a. Determine his or her respiratory rate.	b. Begin assisting his or her breathing

    c. Reevaluate his or her airway status	d. Auscultate his or her breath sounds

13. A palpable pulse is created by:

    a. The pressure of blood against the walls of the arteries.

    b. The pressure that is caused when venous blood returns to the heart

    c. Pressure waves through the arteries caused by cardiac contraction

    d. Electrical conduction in the heart producing ventricular contraction

Section 5 – Patient Assessment

14. Cyanosis of the skin is caused by:

    a. Increased blood oxygen
    b. Peripheral vasodilation
    c. Venous vasoconstriction
    d. Decreased blood oxygen

15. After performing a primary assessment, a rapid scan of the body should be performed in order to:

    a. Determine the need for spinal motion restriction precautions
    b. Identify less obvious injuries that require immediate transport
    c. Look specifically for signs and symptoms of inadequate perfusion
    d. Find and treat injuries or conditions that do not pose a threat to life

16. When assessing a patient's abdomen, you will typically evaluate for all of the following, EXCEPT:

    a. Subcutaneous emphysema
    b. Open wounds or eviscerations
    c. Gross bleeding and tenderness
    d. Rigidity and obvious bleeding

17. As you assess the head of a patient with a suspected spinal injury, your partner should:

    a. Maintain stabilization of the head
    b. Look in the ears for gross bleeding
    c. Prepare the immobilization equipment
    d. Assess the rest of the body for bleeding

18. When interviewing a patient, you can show him or her that you understand the situation by:

    a. repeating statements back to him or her
    b. using medical terminology whenever possible
    c. maintaining constant eye contact
    d. interrupting him or her as needed for clarification

19. Pain which moves from one part of the body to another is _____.

    a. Radiating
    b. Palpating
    c. Provoked
    d. Referred

20. A full body scan should be performed on:

    a. Stable patients
    b. Patients with traumatic injuries
    c. Responsive medical patients and patients without a significant MOI
    d. Patients with a significant MOI and unresponsive medical patients

Section 5 – Patient Assessment

Matching

Match the terms in the first column with the definitions in the second column

SAMPLE

1. _____ S   a. Allergies
2. _____ A   b. Events preceding
3. _____ M   c. Signs / Symptoms
4. _____ P   d. Last oral intake
5. _____ L   e. Medications
6. _____ E   f. Past medical history

OPQRST

1. _____ O   a. Quality of pain
2. _____ P   b. Onset
3. _____ Q   c. Severity
4. _____ R   d. Timing
5. _____ S   e. Provocation
6. _____ T   f. Radiation

DCAP - BTLS

1. _____ D   a. Lacerations
2. _____ C   b. Deformities
3. _____ A   c. Swelling
4. _____ P   d. Punctures / Penetrations
5. _____ B   e. Contusions
6. _____ T   f. Abrasions
7. _____ L   g. Burns
8. _____ S   h. Tenderness

Neurologic Assessment Review Questions – Multiple Choice

1. A neuro exam should be performed as soon as possible on a diver reporting symptoms related to decompression sickness.

    a. True   b. False

2. A neuro examination may need to be performed in a recompression chamber.

    a. True   b. False

3. Recompression of a diver showing signs and symptoms of DCS should be delayed to complete a neuro exam.

    a. True   b. False

4. A neurological examination includes all of the following EXCEPT:

    a. Cranial nerve function   b. Muscle strength check

    c. Sensation check   d. Auscultation of bowel sounds

5. The 12 cranial nerves originate from:

    a. Brain stem   b. Thoracic spine

    c. Optic nerve   d. Cerebrum

6. The Olfactory cranial nerve allows the diver to:

    a. Urinate   b. Speak

    c. Smell   d. Hear

7. Damage to the Oculomotor nerve can cause the affected eye to move down and out.

    a. True   b. False

8. Injury to the Facial nerve can cause signs of a stoke on the effected side.

    a. True   b. False

9. The Glossopharyngeal nerve controls what function?

    a. Swallowing / Gag reflex   b. Tongue movement

    c. Hearing   d. Sensation

10. Tendon reflexes tested during a neuro exam include all of the following EXCEPT:

    a. Knee reflex   b. Ankle reflex

    c. Bicep reflex   d. Wrist reflex

6 Tables – Decompression and Recompression

Diving Tables Review Questions – Multiple Choice

Use the U.S. Navy Tables on pages 79 – 80 for the following questions

1. What is the no-decompression limit for a diver at 47 fsw?

    a. 125 minutes   b. 100 minutes

    c. 92 minutes   d. 74 minutes

2. What is the no-decompression limit for a diver at 93 fsw?

    a. 20 minutes   b. 30 minutes

    c. 25 minutes   d. 39 minutes

3. What repetitive group would a diver be in after spending 42 minutes at 50 fsw?

    a. G   b. F   c. H   d. E

4. What repetitive group would a diver be in after spending 112 minutes at 40 fsw?

    a. K   b. L   c. H   d. M

5. A diver completes a dive with a repetitive group designation of I, the diver remains on the surface for 2 hours and then makes a dive to 60 fsw. What is this diver's residual nitrogen time (RNT)?

    a. 34   b. 40   c. 42   d. 43

6. A diver completes a dive with a repetitive group designation of L, the diver remains on the surface for 2 hours 30 minutes and then makes a dive to 100 fsw. What is this diver's residual nitrogen time (RNT)?

    a. 33   b. 42   c. 38   d. 45

7. What is the 'Repetitive Group Designation' (RNT) for the diver in question 6 following his surface interval?

    a. J   b. I   c. K   d. M

8. A diver has a repetitive group designation of N. How long would this diver need to wait to have a RNT of zero?

    a. 14:06   b. 14:05   c. 13:31   d. 12:37

9. A diver has a repetitive group designation of A. How long would this diver need to wait to have a RNT of zero?

    a. 0:10   b. 2:20   c. 2:21   d. 3:20

Section 6 – Decompression and Recompression

10. A diver completes a dive to 115 fsw with a bottom time of 22 minutes. What is this diver's repetitive group?

    a. K   b. J   c. L   d. M

11. A diver completes a dive to 65 fsw with a bottom time of 45 minutes. After a 2 hour 30 minute surface interval, the diver returns to 45 fsw for 75 minutes. What is the repetitive group designation at the end of the second dive?

    a. O   b. N   c. Z   d. B

12. A diver completes a dive to 45 fsw with a bottom time of 45 minutes. After a 2 hour surface interval, the diver returns to 60 fsw for 75 minutes. What is the repetitive group designation at the end of the second dive?

    a. O   b. N   c. Z   d. B

13. A diver completes a dive to 100 fsw with a bottom time of 30 minutes. After a 1 hour and 45 minute surface interval, the diver returns to 60 fsw for 40 minutes. What is the repetitive group designation at the end of the second dive?

    a. O   b. N   c. Z   d. B

14. A diver completes a dive to 140 fsw with a bottom time of 30 minutes. After a 1 hour and 45 minute surface interval, the diver returns to 60 fsw for 40 minutes. What is the repetitive group designation at the end of the second dive?

    a. O   b. N   c. Z   d. B

15. A normal surface interval for an 'Oxygen Surface Decompression' procedure should not exceed:

    a. 15 minutes   b. 12 minutes   c. 5 minutes   d. 10 minutes

Treatment Tables Review Question – Multiple Choice

Use the US Navy Treatment Tables on Pages 103 - 126.

1. The USN TT6A is currently not recommended to be used in its' original format. What modification to TT6A should be made in the treatment of an arterial gas embolus?

    a. Do not descend to 165 fsw   b. Keep the patient on 100% oxygen

    c. Modify the treatment gas below 60 fsw   d. Never use a USN TT6A

2. What modified treatment gas can be used on both USN TT6A and the COMEX 30 table below 60 fsw?

    a. 50/50 oxygen mix   b. 60% oxygen mix

    c. 30 percent oxygen mix   c. 100 % oxygen mix

3. The standard oxygen period at 60 fsw for the USN treatment tables is:

    a. 25 minutes   b. 30 minutes   c. 20 minutes   d. 60 minutes

Section 6 – Decompression and Recompression

4. The standard patient rate of descent for the USN treatment tables is:

    a. 20 ft/min   b. 30 ft/min   c. 10 ft/min   d. 1 ft/min

5. The standard patient ascent rate for the USN treatment tables is:

    a. 1 ft/min   b. 20 ft/min   c. 10 ft/min   d. 30 ft/min

6. USN TT6 should be used for Type I DCS symptoms when no neurological exam is conducted.

    a. True   b. False

7. Most monoplace chamber may be used for the treatment of a Type II decompression issue.

    a. True   b. False

8. In-water recompression should be used regardless if oxygen as treatment gas is NOT available.

    a. True   b. False

9. The Hawaiian and Australian 'In-Water Recompression' tables both use 100% oxygen at what depth?

    a. 165 fsw   b. 100 fsw   c. 45 fsw   d. 30 fsw

10. All established 'In-Water Recompression' tables require additional oxygen administration on the surface following decompression.

    a. True   b. False

11. USN Oxygen treatment tables may be extended at both 60 fsw and 30 fsw.

    a. True   b. False

12. Oxygen period extensions of USN TT6 may cause which of the following?

    a. Tender DCS   b. Pulmonary toxicity   c. Oxygen seizure   d. All of the above

13. When extending a USN TT6, the tender/medic will be required to breathe 100% oxygen for a longer period of time during ascent to the surface.

    a. True   b. False

14. A tender/medic can routinely start breathing 100% oxygen at 60 fsw.

    a. True   b. False

15. On ascent from treatment depth, arms and legs can be crossed with no concerns?

    a. True   b. False

Section 6 – Decompression and Recompression

7 Hyperbaric Chambers

Hyperbaric Chamber Review Questions – Multiple Choice

1. Hyperbaric chambers are considered 'Pressure Vessels for Human Occupancy' (PVHO) by ASME.

    a. True   b. False

2. ASME stands for the American Society of Mechanical Engineers.

    a. True   b. False

3. The second 'primary' certification organization for hyperbaric chambers is:

    a. NAPA   b. USCG   c. USDA   d. NFPA

4. Besides recompression and decompression chambers, what other items are considered PVHOs?

    a. Diving bells   b. Personnel transfer chambers

    c. Submersibles   d. All of the above

5. To qualify as a PVHO, the vessel must be subjected to at least _____ differential pressure.

    a. 2 psi   b. 14.7 psi   c. 33 psi   d. 33 fsw

6. PVHO-2 addresses which hyperbaric chamber components?

    a. Bulkheads   b. BIBBs   c. Fire suppression systems   d. Acrylic windows

7. The National Fire Protection Association (NFPA), in the US, regulates fire safety requirements for PVHOs.

    a. True   b. False

8. NFPA Chapter 20 is the regulatory standard for all hazards appropriate to Hyperbaric Facilities.

    a. True   b. False

9. Generally speaking, what are the 2 types of hyperbaric chambers.

    a. Monoplace / Multiplace   b. Deck decompression / portable

    c. Portable / Submersible   d. Human / animal

10. Portable, emergency chambers, such as the SOS Hyperlite, are only capable of 2 ATA during the transport of an injured diver.

    a. True   b. False

11. With regards to fire safety in the hyperbaric chamber, which items are NOT allowed in the chamber?

    a. Cellular telephones   b. Hand warmers

    c. Newspapers   d. All of the above

Section 7 – Hyperbaric Chambers

12. At 6 ATA, a chamber fire will burn at the same force and rate as a(n) _____ oxygen mix at the surface?

    a. 40 %   b. 20 %   c. 80%   d. 100%

13. The primary goal of chamber fire safety is to:

    a. Check the extinguishers   b. Install a deluge system

    c. Prevent fires   d. None of the above

14. The Apollo One fire was considered to be a hyperbaric fire.

    a. True   b. False

15. NFPA 701 requires that all patient and tender clothing be 100% cotton.

    a. True   b. False

16. Deluge and sprinkler fire systems are mandatory in Class A multiplace chamber in the US.

    a. True   b. False

17. What type of compressors can be used to pressurize and operate a PVHO?

    a. High pressure / low pressure   b. Intrinsically safe

    c. Braun / Deere   d. Nitrogen / Helium

18. Volume tanks associated with a hyperbaric chamber should be of sufficient size to pressurize the chamber to 6 ATA within _____ minutes.

    a. 10   b. 15   c. 5   d. 8.5

19. Air supplies to the chamber should be filtered to at least Grade _____ SCUBA air quality.

    a. B   b. E   c. F   d. G

20. The standard treatment gas for USN Treatment Tables at 60 fsw is:

    a. 50/50 heliox   b. Trimix   c. 100% oxygen   d. None of the above

21. Delivery systems for treatment gases into a PVHO can utilize quarter turn 'ball' valves.

    a. True   b. False

22. The rapid opening of gas line valves can cause adiabatic heating.

    a. True   b. False

23. The acronym, 'BIBS' stands for:

    a. Blonde in blue shorts   b. Built in breathing system

    c. Bars in Bay Shore   d. None of the above

Section 7 – Hyperbaric Chambers

24. What gas is delivered via the BIBS?

    a. Exhaust gas   b. Nitrogen   c. Treatment   d. Ventilation

25. The 'Overboard' dump system allows what gas to be exhausted from the chamber?

    a. Patient exhaled gas   b. Oxygen   c. Chamber air   d. Nitrogen

26. A standard BIBS consists of how many hose lines?

    a. 1   b. 2   c. 3   d. 4

27. Correct application of the BIBS is important to prevent:

    a. Leaking of oxygen and increasing the PPO_2 of the ambient chamber air

    b. The patient from breathing the treatment gas

    c. The patient from talking

    d. Wasting oxygen

28. PVHO should be equipped with the following equipment?

    a. Atmospheric monitor   b. Depth gauges   c. Temperature monitors   d. All of the above

29. Hyperbaric chambers should have communications systems so the operator and medic can communicate. In the event of communication system failure, what backup system can be used?

    a. Sign language   b. Morse code   c. Smoke signals   d. SCUBA hand signals

30. All ancillary equipment must be certified for hyperbaric chamber use with no modification.

    a. True   b. False

31. Chamber air must not be allowed to rise over _____ oxygen content during treatment runs.

    a. 25%   b. 19%   c. 20.7%   d. 50%

Section 7 – Hyperbaric Chambers

Find the Terms

B	I	B	S	W	N	H	F	Q	T	W	M	Y	B	R
L	W	O	W	B	F	N	T	P	V	H	O	H	U	E
M	U	L	T	I	P	L	A	C	E	T	N	N	L	C
O	T	T	G	H	A	P	S	O	N	H	I	R	K	O
N	I	T	R	O	X	O	C	M	T	I	T	M	H	M
O	X	Y	G	E	N	R	E	P	J	O	O	T	E	P
P	O	E	K	G	U	T	N	R	L	P	R	A	A	R
A	S	M	E	J	T	A	D	E	S	C	E	N	D	E
L	C	H	E	C	K	L	I	S	T	C	J	W	E	S
E	E	L	O	W	P	R	E	S	S	U	R	E	R	S
S	C	R	U	B	B	E	R	O	M	V	A	L	V	E
K	D	A	H	I	G	H	P	R	E	S	S	U	R	E
H	U	M	I	D	I	T	Y	S	D	E	L	U	G	E
C	A	R	B	O	N	M	O	N	O	X	I	D	E	L
H	Y	P	E	R	L	I	T	E	D	G	T	Y	I	L

Monoplace	Ascend
Multiplace	Descend
Hyperlite	Scrubber
Oxygen	Recompress
ASME	PVHO
Carbon Monoxide	Monitor
High Pressure	Humidity
Low Pressure	Deluge
Nitrox	Checklist
BIBS	Portal
NFPA	Bulkhead
Vent	Valve
Monoplace	Ascend
Multiplace	Descend
Hyperlite	Scrubber

8 Pressure Injuries / Illness

Fill In the Blanks

Label the appropriate anatomical structure using the terms to the left.

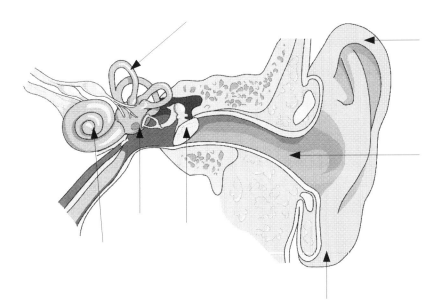

a. Pinna

b. External canal

c. Targus

d. Tympanic membrane

e. Round window

f. Semi-circular canals

g. Cochlea

Pressure Injuries and Illness Review Questions – Multiple Choice

1. Injuries caused by increase or decrease of pressure are called?

    a. Barotrauma   b. Decompression sickness

    c. Penetrating trauma   d. Pressure trauma

2. Solid organs affected by pressure changes include:

    a. liver   b. Spleen   c. Soft tissue   d. None of the above

3. Hollow organs or gas containing spaces in the body are at risk of barotrauma:

    a. During ventilation   b. Only during ascent

    c. Only on descent   d. During any pressure change

4. The most common barotrauma injury in the hyperbaric environment is:

    a. Gastric distention   b. Pulmonary barotrauma

    c. Middle ear barotrauma   d. Suit squeeze

Section 8 – Pressure Injuries / Illness

5. Outer ear barotrauma is not possible in a hyperbaric chamber.

    a. True   b. False

6. The greatest likelihood for middle ear trauma is during descent from:

    a. 30 fsw to 60 fsw   b. 60 fsw to 100 fsw   c. Surface to 10 fsw   d. Any ascent

7. The anatomical structure which equalizes the middle ear is the:

    a. Chest tube   b. Bronchi   c. Eustachian tubes   d. Sinuses

8. While operating a hyperbaric chamber, the patient begins to complain of middle ear pain. The best course of action is to:

    a. Continue the descent   b. Speed up the descent

    c. Slow the descent   d. Stop the descent

9. What injury is risked with aggressive Valsalva maneuvers in the chamber?

    a. Bleeding in the eyes   b. Pneumothorax

    c. Round window rupture   d. Incontinence

10. A buildup of Cerumen (ear wax) in the external ear canal may lead to an infectious condition known as:

    a. Ruptured tympanic membrane   b. Otitis Externa

    c. Athletes foot   d. Vertigo

11. Gastrointestinal barotrauma can be caused by swallowing air or gas during a hyperbaric treatment. When would this condition be most pronounced?

    a. At the surface   b. 60 fsw to 30 fsw   c. 30 fsw to Surface   d. At 165 fsw

12. A sinus block on descent may be relieved by an aggressive Valsalva maneuver.

    a. True   b. False

13. A reverse sinus block occurs when the sinus congest while at depth.

    a. True   b. False

14. Tooth squeeze can be caused by the following.

    a. A cracked tooth   b. Loose fillings

    c. A cavity in the tooth d. All of the above

15. Mask squeeze is caused by not equalizing the pressure inside the facemask while diving.

    a. True   b. False

Section 8 – Pressure Injuries / Illness

16. Underwater blast effect is greater than on land or in the air because:

    a. Air is more dense
    b. The effect is the same
    c. Water is non-compressible
    d. Water is compressible

17. Regarding underwater blast injuries, the injuries will be more severe because underwater the pressure wave is transmitted through the body unlike an air blast where the pressure wave is reflected off the body surface.

    a. True
    b. False

18. A diver holding his breath underwater and ascending is at risk of which of the following?

    a. Pulmonary barotrauma
    b. Subcutaneous emphysema
    c. Arterial gas embolus
    d. All of the above

19. The physical law which addresses pulmonary barotrauma is:

    a. Dalton's Law
    b. Murphy's Law
    c. Henry's Law
    d. Boyle's Law

20. What anatomical structure in the lungs is damaged in pulmonary over-inflation injury?

    a. Bronchi
    b. Bronchioles
    c. Trachea
    d. Alveoli

21. A pneumothorax is best described as:

    a. Air escaping the lung into the pleural space
    b. A shift of the injured lung
    c. A deviated trachea
    d. Air in the soft tissues

22. In a hyperbaric chamber, pulmonary barotrauma may occur during:

    a. Ascent
    b. Descent
    c. At treatment depth
    d. None of the above

23. A pneumothorax may develop into a more serious condition known as a:

    a. Myocardial infarct
    b. Tension pneumothorax
    c. Pulmonary embolus
    d. Pneumonia

24. Initial treatment for a pneumothorax is:

    a. High flow oxygen
    b. Aspirin
    c. Chest tube insertion
    d. Thoracic decompression

25. Treatment for a tension pneumothorax includes:

    a. Thoracic decompression over the effected side
    b. Administration of Hartman solution
    c. Valsalva maneuver
    d. Rapid ascent

26. Signs and symptoms of an arterial gas embolus (AGE) will present within _____ minute of surfacing?

    a. 15 minutes
    b. 30 minutes
    c. 60 minutes
    d. 8 hours

Section 8 – Pressure Injuries / Illness

27. The signs and symptoms of an AGE are similar to what other medical condition?

    a. Heart attack   b. Pneumonia   c. Sepsis   d. Cerebral vascular accident

28. Immediate treatment for an AGE include:

    a. Immediate recompression on a modified USN TT6A   b. High flow oxygen

    c. Rehydration (IV) therapy   d. All of the above

29. Other signs and symptoms of an arterial gas embolus may include:

    a. Confusion   b. Altered mental status   c. Dizziness/headache   d. All of the above

30. The uploading of inert gas molecules into the tissues and blood stream of a diver is a function of which physical law?

    a. Boyle's Law   b. Dalton's Law   c. Charles' Law   d. Henry's Law

31. Who is credited with developing the first decompression tables for divers?

    a. Haldane   b. Dr. Kindwall   c. Dr. End   d. Boyle

32. During ascent, a diver must make 'deco' stops to allow for:

    a. On-gassing   b. Off-gassing   c. Saturation   d. Hydrating

33. If a diver returns to the surface before decompressing, _____ can be formed in the tissues and bloodstream.

    a. Micro-nuclei   b. Bubbles   c. Oxygen   d. None of the above

34. Which diving gas is most like to increase the risk of decompression sickness in a diver who spends 20 minutes at 100 fsw?

    a. Nitrox   b. Trimix   c. Heliox   d. Air

35. A patent foramen ovale (PFO) is found in the septum separating the atria of the heart. This abnormality in divers can cause what to happen?

    a. Inert gas bubbles will not pass through the opening

    b. Inert gas bubbles can pass from the venous system to the arterial system

    c. Extravascular bubbles will always stay on the venous side

    d. Inert gas bubbles can pass from the arterial system directly into the venous system

36. The danger of a PFO is that if inert gas bubbles enter the arterial side of the circulatory system, they can cause an AGE and will become lodged downstream in the system.

    a. True   b. False

37. Type I decompression sickness is often described as "pain-only' DCS.

    a. True   b. False

Section 8 – Pressure Injuries / Illness

38. Type II decompression sickness (DCS) involves some insult to the central nervous system.

    a. True   b. False

39. Many of the signs and symptoms of Type II DCS are similar to flu-like symptoms.

    a. True   b. False

40. The MAJORITY of DCS injured divers will present for treatment within _____ hour(s).

    a. 24 hours   b. 48 hours   c. 1 hour   d. 8 hours

41. Initial field care by the diver medic prior to reaching the hyperbaric chamber would be to:

    a. Provide 100% high-flow oxygen   b. Hydrate the diver

    c. Use gentle handing techniques while moving the diver   d. All of the above

42. The inert gas bubbles will _____ in size when pressure is increased in a hyperbaric chamber.

    a. Increase   b. Decrease   c. Stay the same   d. Dissolve

43. Decompression sickness can occur at any point during a dive.

    a. True   b. False

44. The off-gassing process of Inert gas bubbles is function of the :

    a. Lungs   b. Kidneys   c. Heart   d. Spleen

45. A diver flying in a commercial aircraft immediately following a dive is at greater risk of a DCS hit.

    a. True   b. False

Section 8 – Pressure Injuries / Illness

Find the Terms

B	A	R	O	T	R	A	U	M	A	E	F	G	T	D	O	H	N	T	L
R	S	C	O	C	H	L	E	A	B	P	A	R	A	L	Y	S	I	S	E
A	D	F	T	Y	U	I	O	N	D	I	F	F	U	S	I	O	N	W	U
D	E	H	Y	D	R	A	T	I	O	N	W	A	T	Y	U	L	C	N	K
Y	A	R	T	E	R	I	A	L	E	M	B	O	L	I	S	M	U	M	O
C	E	R	U	M	E	N	C	B	Y	K	E	V	I	T	I	A	T	P	C
A	A	A	W	A	T	E	L	L	E	D	N	A	B	Y	N	L	A	U	Y
R	R	Q	A	S	P	I	R	I	N	U	D	L	L	P	U	A	N	M	T
D	R	I	N	K	W	A	T	E	R	S	S	E	T	E	S	I	E	O	E
I	A	W	E	F	P	F	O	K	N	R	E	X	C	O	G	S	O	I	R
A	T	P	N	E	U	M	O	T	H	O	R	A	X	N	R	E	U	R	H
S	R	T	S	I	L	E	N	T	B	U	B	B	L	E	T	Y	S	U	O
S	I	N	U	S	M	W	A	N	X	I	E	T	Y	Q	T	U	K	L	T
Q	G	E	Y	P	O	L	Y	P	B	R	W	C	E	R	E	B	R	A	L
U	E	I	O	U	N	A	P	U	L	M	O	N	A	R	Y	D	O	H	W
E	R	E	G	J	A	D	H	B	G	S	O	X	Y	G	E	N	T	E	H
E	W	O	V	E	R	P	R	E	S	S	U	R	I	Z	A	T	I	O	N
Z	G	K	S	S	Y	P	A	R	A	S	T	H	E	S	I	A	J	E	D
E	M	B	O	L	I	S	M	T	Y	P	E	T	W	O	D	H	R	S	D
V	E	S	T	I	B	U	L	A	R	N	E	U	R	O	L	O	G	I	C

Pneumothorax	Type two	Triger
Barotrauma	Embolism	Ovale
Cochlea	Pulmonary	PFO
Bradycardia	Cerebral	Malaise
Dehydration	Overpressurization	Paresthesia
Cerumen	Leukocyte	Paralysis
Vestibular	Diffusion	Anxiety
Squeeze	Silent bubble	Cutaneous
Mask	Pol	Neurologic
Drink water	Wattelle	Oxygen
Type one	Bert	Aspirin
Bends	Moir	Sinus

9 Environmental and Marine Injuries

Medical Review Questions – Multiple Choice

1. Defined, hypothermia is the _____ of the core body temperature _____ normal temperatures.

    a. Reduction / below   b. Reduction / above   c. Increase / above   d. Increase / below

2. Blue lips and/or blue fingertips in the hypothermic patient are due to:

    a. Frost bite   b. Contusions   c. Blood vessel constriction   d. Trench foot

3. Shivering is a way for the body to generate heat in a hypothermic patient.

    a. True   b. False

4. Localized cold injuries include all of the following EXCEPT:

    a. Trench foot   b. Frost Nip   c. Frost bite   d. Apnea

5. Frost bite involves the actual freezing of body tissue.

    a. True   b. False

6. Contributing factor for trench foot, or immersion foot, are all of the following except:

    a. Cold environment   b. Wet environment   c. No way to dry or warm feet   d. Dry environment

7. Frost nip is the superficial partial freezing of the epidermal tissues.

    a. True   b. False

8. Removal of jewelry and constricting clothing is important for a frostbite patient because it can reduce circulation in swollen tissues.

    a. True   b. False

9. Passive and active rewarming is required for frostbitten tissue.

    a. True   b. False

10. Hyperthermia is the _____ of the core body temperature (CBT) _____ the normal temperature range.

    a. Increase / above   b. Increase / below   c. Decrease / below   d. Decrease / above

11. Signs and symptoms of heat exhaustion include all of the following EXCEPT:

    a. Moist skin   b. Cool, pale skin   c. Headache   d. Dry, hot skin

12. Heat stroke is a life threatening injury in which the body has lost the ability to regulate its body temperature.

    a. True   b. False

Section 9 – Environmental and Marine Injuries

13. A heat stroke victim requires immediate external cooling, include ice packs placed in the groin, arm pits, and around the neck.

    a. True   b. False

14. Drowning is caused by a series of events that ultimately lead to panic and inhalation of water.

    a. True   b. False

15. Near drowning is a condition by which the diver has survived a 'drowning' incident, but survives for at least _____ hours.

    a. 12   b. 8   c. 24   d. 36

16. During the recovery time for a near drowning incident, the victim is susceptible to death due to damage to the _____ system.

    a. Cardiovascular   b. Respiratory   c. Endocrine   d. Neurological

17. Shallow water blackout is caused when _____ is metabolized and pressure is _____.

    a. Oxygen / reduced   b. Nitrogen / reduced   c. Oxygen / increased   d. Nitrogen / increased

18. Anaphylaxis is a severe allergic reaction to something in the environment.

    a. True   b. False

19. Immediate treatment for life threatening anaphylaxis includes:

    a. 0.3 mg epinephrine IM   b. High flow oxygen   c. Diphenhydramine 50mg   d. All of the above

20. Wounds received due to marine animals or organisms have a high rate of infection.

    a. True   b. False

21. All wounds caused by marine trauma should be _____ as soon as possible.

    a. Sutured   b. Bandaged   c. Irrigated   d. None of the above

22. Administration of antibiotic as a prophylactic measure is acceptable in cases of a marine trauma.

    a. True   b. False

23. Attacks by large marine animals should be treated the same as significant trauma incidents.

    a. True   b. False

24. A priority, following an traumatic attack by a shark, should be all of the following EXCEPT:

    a. Stop the bleeding   b. Maintain airway & breathing   c. Treat for shock   d. Call animal rescue

25. Envenomations by marine animals can cause life-threatening injuries. The diver medic should concentration on support of the patient's vital functions in this event.

    a. True   b. False

Section 9 – Environmental and Marine Injuries

26. Neurotoxin envenomations attack which body system?

    a. Respiratory   b. Cardiac   c. Central nervous   d. Endocrine

27. For many stings and bite in the marine environment, the only definitive treatment is:

    a. Cold water immersion   b. Rotating tourniquets

    c. Antivenom   d. Heat packs applied to the wound

28. Many sea jelly wounds may be treated with hot water / vinegar compresses.

    a. True   b. False

Find the Terms

H	Y	P	O	T	H	E	R	M	I	C	F	T	J	R
Y	W	C	E	R	U	M	E	N	R	M	M	A	K	O
P	V	C	B	L	A	C	K	O	U	T	F	D	R	Q
O	O	O	T	I	T	I	S	E	X	T	E	R	N	A
T	M	F	R	O	S	T	B	I	T	E	J	O	K	N
H	I	R	O	C	T	O	P	U	S	Q	Y	W	X	A
E	T	O	M	O	R	A	Y	E	E	L	F	N	H	P
R	I	S	L	N	O	W	H	I	T	E	T	I	P	H
M	N	T	R	Y	K	S	F	E	T	H	J	N	K	Y
I	G	N	D	S	E	A	S	I	C	K	R	G	M	L
A	B	I	N	F	E	C	T	I	O	N	L	G	R	A
I	F	P	R	O	M	E	T	H	A	Z	I	N	E	X
G	R	E	A	T	W	H	I	T	E	G	O	Y	E	I
E	S	E	A	S	N	A	K	E	S	F	N	U	F	S
S	R	L	R	S	C	O	R	P	I	O	N	Y	I	B

Hypothermic	Infection
Hypothermia	Mako
Hyperthermia	Reef
Heatstroke	Great white
Frostbite	Whitetip
Cerumen	Eel
Drowning	Moray eel
Blackout	Octopus
Seasick	Sea snakes
Vomiting	Lion
Anaphylaxis	Scorpion
Promethazine	Infection
Hypothermic	Mako
Hypothermia	Reef
Hyperthermia	Great white

10 Airway and Breathing

Medical Review Questions – Multiple Choice

1. What is the average oxygen delivery percentage of a pocket mask connected to a 15L/min flow?

    a. up to 55%   b. 20-30%   c. 30-40%   d. 100%

2. A complete non-rebreather oxygen mask will deliver _____ % of oxygen at a 15L/min flow.

    a. 70-75%   b. 90-100%   c. 20-30%   d. 55%

3. Flow restricted pressure/demand delivery devices work best on which patients?

    a. Obese   b. Conscious   c. Unconscious   d. Intubated

4. The Bag-Valve-Mask (BVM) is sealed to the patients' face using what grip?

    a. Full face   b. Kung Fu   c. E-C   d. Q-A

5. The BVM has both a(n) _____ supply hose and a(n) _____ reservoir bag.

    a. air / oxygen   b. air / air   c. oxygen / oxygen   d. oxygen / air

6. Flow restricted pressure/demand delivery devices pressure relief will activate at _____ cm H_2O.

    a. 50   b. 40   c. 30   d. 100

7. Oropharyngeal airways (OPA) are designed to prevent the _____ from blocking the upper airway.

    a. Tongue   b. Epiglottis   c. Teeth   d. Nasal passage

8. Contraindications for insertion of an OPA include:

    a. Conscious patient   b. Active gag reflex   c. Both a & b   d. None of the above

9. If the patient regains a gag reflex, the OPA should be removed.

    a. True   b. False

10. The OPA is sized by measuring the device:

    a. Corner of mouth to earlobe   b. Corner of the nostril to corner of the mouth

    c. Corner of mouth to the pinna   d. Tip of the nose to mouth

11. In removing the OPA, the diver medic should:

    a. Rotate the airway 180°   b. Rotate the airway 90°

    c. Follow anatomical curve   d. Pull the airway straight up

Section 10 – Airway and Breathing

12. Nasopharyngeal airways (NPA) may be used on _____ patients.

    a. Conscious   b. Active gag reflex   c. Unconscious   d. All of the above

13. The NPA is sized by measuring the device:

    a. Corner of the nostril to earlobe   b. Corner of the nostril to corner of the mouth

    c. Corner of mouth to the pinna   d. Tip of the nose to mouth

14. Contraindications to the use of a NPA include:

    a. Head injury   b. Facial trauma   c. Nasal blood drainage   d. All of the above

15. Orotracheal suction devices include:

    a. Manual   b. Portable   c. Mounted   d. All of the above

16. Orotracheal suctioning is used to remove _____ from a patient's airway.

    a. Blood   b. Vomit   c. Clotting blood   d. All of the above

17 Suction should not be applied for more than _____ seconds.

    a. 5   b. 10   c. 15   d. 20

18. When inserting a suction catheter into the patient's mouth, suction at the tip should be active.

    a. True   b. False

19. When using a bulb syringe aspirator (turkey baster), the bulb should be _____ during insertion.

    a. Compressed   b. Decompressed   c. Inflated   d. None of the above

20. The suction catheter is measured from the _____ to the _____ .

    a. Corner of mouth to earlobe   b. Corner of the nostril to corner of the mouth

    c. Corner of mouth to the pinna   d. Tip of the nose to mouth

21. Many advanced airways used by diver medics are called "blind insertion" airways, which means what?

    a. Trachea must be visualized   b. No manual airway maneuver is performed

    c. No visualization of the upper airway is required   d. A laryngoscope must be used

22. The "Esophageal Tracheal Combitube" (ETC) is correctly inserted into the patient's _____.

    a. Trachea   b. Larynx   c. Esophagus   d. Lungs

23. The ETC is constructed with a double lumen. This allows the airway to still function in event that it is inserted into the patient's _____.

    a. Trachea   b. Larynx   c. Esophagus   d. Lungs

24. Initial ventilations on an inserted ETC should be attempted on which tube?

    a. #1 / Blue   b. #2 Blue   c. #1 Clear   d. #2 Clear

Section 10 – Airway and Breathing

25. The standard sized ETC is limited to patients who are _____ to _____ feet tall.

    a. 4 / 5　　　b. 5 / 6　　　c. 6 / 7　　　d. Infants

26. The ETC SA (small adult) is designed to be used on patients who are _____ to _____ feet tall.

    a. 4 / 5　　　b. 5 / 6　　　c. 6 / 7　　　d. Infants

27. In reference to the KING LTS-D airway, selecting the inappropriate size tube could cause intubation of the patients' _____.

    a. Trachea　　　b. Larynx　　　c. Esophagus　　　d. Lungs

28. The KING LTS-D airways are available in several sizes based on the patients' height. A size #3 airway would be appropriate for a patient _____ to _____ feet tall.

    a. 4 / 5　　　b. 5 / 6　　　c. 6 / 7　　　d. Infants

29. For a 6 foot tall patient, which size KING LTS-D airway would be appropriate?

    a. #3　　　b. #4　　　c. #5　　　d. #2

30. Insertion of an endotracheal tube (ETT) normally requires additional skills and equipment to perform.

    a. True　　　b. False

31. Blind insertion of an endotracheal tube (ETT) can be accomplished by using what type of adjunct airway?

    a. Oropharyngeal　　　b. Nasopharyngeal　　　c. S.A.L.T.　　　d. ETC

32. A stylet is used with an ETT to assist in _____.

    a. Removal　　　b. Securing the ETT　　　c. Insertion　　　d. Operation

33. When using a laryngoscope to insert an ETT, what anatomical structure is the diver medic looking for?

    a. Vocal cords　　　b. Epiglottis　　　c. Carina　　　d. Tongue

34. The Laryngeal Mask Airway (LMA) is a single cuff airway designed to be placed where?

    a. Nasopharynx　　　b. Esophagus　　　c. Larynx　　　d. Trachea

35. The LMA completely control the airway to prevent aspiration of stomach contents.

    a. True　　　b. False

36. The LMA is correctly sized by using the patients' _____ as a guide.

    a. Height　　　b. Weight　　　c. Neck size　　　d. Finger size

37. Any surgical airway procedure by the diver medic should only be attempted after _____ has failed.

    a. Manual airway opening procedures　　　b. Manual ventilations

    c. Invasive airway insertion　　　d. All of the above

Section 10 – Airway and Breathing

38. Sterile technique should be practiced when performing surgical airway procedures.

    a. True	b. False

39. A 14 gauge 2 inch IV catheter is a viable alternative to a surgical airway.

    a. True	b. False

40. Naso- and orogastric tubes are used to decompress which organ?

    a. Bladder	b. Large intestine	c. Stomach	d. Lungs

41. Nasogastric tubes are measured from the _____, over the ear, and to the base of the _____.

    a. Mouth / stomach	b. Nose / sternum	c. Nose / stomach	d. Mouth / stomach

Identify the Airways

a. _____	b. _____

c. _____	d. _____

e. _____	f. _____

Section 10 – Airway and Breathing

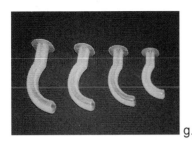 g. _____ 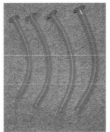 h. _____

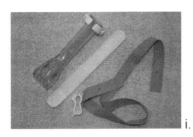 i. _____ 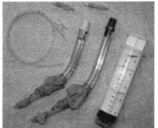 j. _____

Fill In The Blanks

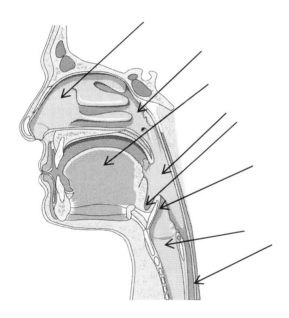

a. Epiglottis

b. Trachea

c. Esophagus

d. Nasal passage

e. Tongue

f. Oropharynx

g. Vallecula

h. Nasopharynx

Section 10 – Airway and Breathing

Find the Terms

O	R	O	P	H	A	R	Y	N	G	E	A	L	F	L
F	S	H	L	Y	P	L	M	A	J	E	Y	N	P	A
E	U	K	A	P	N	M	A	S	K	S	Y	E	H	R
W	C	E	R	O	I	N	L	O	X	Y	G	E	N	Y
N	T	C	Y	X	A	E	H	P	K	R	A	N	E	N
A	I	O	N	I	C	A	O	H	R	I	V	D	E	G
S	O	M	G	C	R	C	P	A	P	N	E	O	D	O
O	N	B	E	Q	I	Y	A	R	S	G	W	T	L	S
G	T	I	A	Y	C	T	W	Y	T	E	A	R	E	C
A	I	T	L	E	O	K	I	N	G	N	V	A	C	O
S	P	U	M	L	I	R	E	G	T	L	E	C	R	P
T	W	B	S	I	D	R	Y	E	R	U	F	H	I	E
R	W	E	A	S	P	I	R	A	T	E	O	I	C	I
I	S	R	L	U	N	G	S	L	E	Y	R	A	T	D
C	Q	M	T	R	A	C	H	E	A	T	M	L	P	S

Oropharyngeal

Nasopharyngeal

Oxygen

BSI

Trachea

Endotracheal

Laryngoscope

CPAP

Aspirate

Laryngeal

Combitube

King

LMA

Syringe

Needle cric

Cricoid

Waveform

Lungs

Suction tip

Mask

OPA

NPA

Hypoxic

11 Vascular Access and Medication Administration

Fill In The Blanks

Identify the Six Patient "Rights" as they pertain to medical administration

1. _____

2. _____

3. _____

4. _____

5. _____

6. _____

Match the Routes of Administration

Percutaneous Route_____

Enteral Route_____

Parenteral Route_____

a. Intravenous
b. Intramuscular
c. Intraossious
d. Transcutaneous
e. Sublingual
f. Subcutaneous
g. Oral

Use These Formulas for the Next Section

Medication Concentration On Hand Calculation
$$\text{concentration on hand (mg/ml)} = \frac{\text{weight on hand (mg)}}{\text{volume on hand (ml)}}$$

Section 11 – Vascular Access and Medication Administration

Calculate the Concentration On Hand.

1. A 50ml multidose vial of 2% Lidocaine containing 20mg/ml concentration. Calculate the concentration on hand.

2. A 2ml preloaded syringe of Narcan contains 1mg/ml concentration. Calculate the concentration on hand.

3. A 10ml preload of Atropine Sulfate contains 0.1mg/ml concentration. Calculate the concentration on hand.

Volume To Be Administered

$$\text{volume to be administered (ml)} = \frac{\text{volume on hand (ml)} \times \text{desired dose (mg)}}{\text{weight on hand (mg)}}$$

---

1. The DMO orders 5mg of Valium to sedate a patient. A multidose vial is available which contains a concentration of 40mg in 10ml. Calculate amount to be administered to the patient.

2. The DMO orders 4mg of Narcan to counter act a morphine injection. 2ml preloaded syringes of Narcan are available in a concentration of 1mg/ml. Calculate the amount to be administered to the patient.

Section 11 – Vascular Access and Medication Administration

Intravenous / Intraosseous Drip Rate Formula
drops per minute (gtt/min) = $\dfrac{\text{total amount of fluid to be administered (ml) x drop factor (gtt/min)}}{\text{total time in minutes}}$

1. The DMO orders an infusion rate of 300ml/hr via an intravenous line. Calculate the drip rate per minute.

2. The DMO orders an infusion rate of 500ml/hr via an intravenous line. Calculate the drip rate per minute.

3. The DMO orders an infusion rate of 100ml/hr via an intravenous line. Calculate the drip rate per minute.

Section 11 – Vascular Access and Medication Administration

Review Questions – Multiple Choice

1. A diver medic is authorized to administer medications by _____

    a. The Company   b. IMCA   c. NBDHMT   d. the Diving Medical Officer

2. Percutaneous administered drugs enter the patient via what mechanism?

    a. Skin   b. Mucus membranes   c. Sublingual   d. All of the above

3. Sublingual medications are administrated typically how?

    a. Under the tongue   b. Between cheek and gums   c. Orally   d. Injection

4. Vital signs must be taken before and after administration of any drug.

    a. True   b. False

5. A subcutaneous injection is administered how?

    a. Short needle / 90°   b. Long needle / 45°   c. Long needle / 90°   d. Short needle / 45°

6. An intramuscular injection is administered how?

    a. Short needle / 90°   b. Long needle / 45°   c. Long needle / 90°   d. Short needle / 45°

7. Prior to administration of a drug, the diver medic must confirm what?

    a. Rule of 9's   b. AVPU scale   c. 6 Patient Rights   d. Injection site

8. An intravenous catheter is inserted where?

    a. Vein   b. Artery   c. Capillary   d. Bone marrow

9. An Intraossious injection is placed into anatomical space/structure?

    a. Vein   b. Artery   c. Capillary   d. Bone marrow

10. When drawing medications from a multidose vial, the diver medic should _____ to facilitate the removal of the medication into the syringe.

    a. Shake the vial   b. Remove the stopper   c. Invert the vial   d. Inject air

11. When drawing medication from an ampule, the diver medic should use what type of needle?

    a. Intraossious   b. Filtered   c. Small gauge   d. Brunard

12. The normal limit of medication injection via the intramuscular route in the thigh is _____ ml.

    a. 1ml   b. 2ml   c. 4ml   d. 5ml

13. The most rapid route for medication absorption is _____.

    a. IV/IO   b. SubQ   c. IM   d. Sublingual

14. Subcutaneous method of injection is used to inject a *maximum* of _____ ml.

    a. 2ml   b. 4ml   c. 10ml   d. 1ml

Section 11 – Vascular Access and Medication Administration

15. Preloaded medication syringes are most frequently used during _____ emergencies.

    a. Cardiac   b. Trauma   c. Environmental   d. Diving

16. Diphenhydramine (Benadryl) is a(n) _____.

    a. Vasoconstrictor   b. Anti-histamine   c. Vasodilator   d. Cardiac medication

17. Epinephrine (adrenalin) is used primarily by the diver medic in life-threatening cases of _____.

    a. Anaphylaxis   b. Diabetes   c. Chest pain   d. COPD

18. The standard adult dose of epinephrine for the medical issue in Question 17 is _____.

    a. 0.5 mg   b. 0.15 mg   c. 0.1 mg   d. 0.3 mg

19. Albuterol (Proventil) is indicated for patients who are experiencing _____.

    a. Chest pain   b. Asthma   c. Angina   d. Headaches

20. Anytime a diver medic is ordered by the DMO to administer morphine sulfate, he/she must also have what drug available?

    a. Valium   b. Narcan   c. Lasix   d. Lidocaine

21. Glucagon is used primarily for _____ patients.

    a. Cardiac   b. Respiratory   c. Diabetic   d. Drowning

22. Lactated Ringers solution is IV fluid of choice for _____ in a _____ patient.

    a. Volume expansion / trauma   b. Volume expansion / drowning

    c. TKO / medical   d. None of these

23. An IV of Normal Saline is normally started to provide _____.

    a. Route for medications   b. Rehydration

    c. Maintain systemic pressure   d. All of the above

24. Oxygen is a flammable gas.

    a. True   b. False

25. Nitroglycerin will cause coronary arteries to _____.

    a. Dilate   b. Constrict   c. Spasm   d. Become more pliable

Section 11 – Vascular Access and Medication Administration

Mix and Match

Column 1

1. Vial _____
2. Metered Dose Inhaler_____
3. Ampule_____
4. Hypodermic Needle_____
5. Intraosseous Device_____
6. Intravenous Catheter_____
7. Barrel_____
8. Pre-loaded Syringe_____
9. IV Administration Set_____
10. Nebulizer_____

Column 2

a. A glass container normally 1 ml
b. A glass container containing larger quantities of a drug
c. The line between the IV bag and cannula
d. Device used to aerosolize medications
e. Medication container of a syringe
f. Pump container containing medication
g. Working end of a syringe
h. A cannula inserted through the bone
i. A cannula inserted into a vein
j. Syringe containing a pre-measure amount of medication

Find the Terms

D	T	P	R	I	N	T	R	A	V	E	N	O	U	S
P	H	A	R	M	A	C	O	L	O	G	Y	H	O	U
K	E	R	G	P	E	R	R	E	C	T	U	M	D	B
V	N	E	N	T	E	R	A	L	D	G	J	P	E	L
O	I	N	J	E	C	T	L	D	A	R	M	U	L	I
I	N	T	R	A	O	S	S	E	O	U	S	L	T	N
M	A	A	R	G	J	C	N	E	E	D	L	E	O	G
P	E	R	C	U	T	A	N	E	O	U	S	X	I	U
F	V	A	G	F	A	S	T	I	O	K	Y	F	D	A
M	I	L	L	I	L	I	T	E	R	D	R	I	P	L
C	A	T	H	E	T	E	R	T	W	P	I	L	L	K
D	L	F	B	I	G	I	O	W	W	R	N	E	T	J
O	D	G	H	J	L	S	U	B	Q	S	G	G	T	S
S	T	E	R	N	U	M	T	A	B	L	E	T	T	M
E	M	A	C	R	O	S	E	T	G	P	E	Z	I	O

Pharmacology	FAST IO
Parenteral	Ampule
Enteral	Vial
Oral	Needle
Percutaneous	Catheter
Per rectum	Dose
CPR	Route
Intraosseous	Drip
Inject	Sublingual
Intravenous	SubQ
Milliliter	KVO
GGT	Tablet
EZ IO	BIG IO
Sternum	Deltoid
Pill	Macroset

Section 12 – Soft Tissue Injuries

12 Soft Tissue Injury

Fill In The Blanks

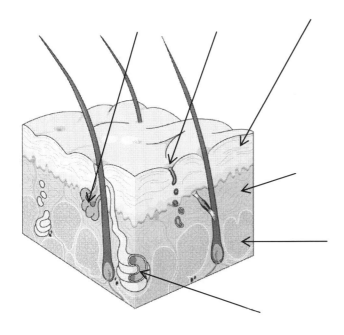

a. Epidermis

b. Dermis

c. Subcutaneous tissue

d. Eccrine gland

e. Sebaceous gland

f. Pore

Mix and Match

Match Column 1 with the correct definition in Column 2

Column 1	Column 2
1. Abrasion	a.___ Cut inflicted by a sharp object
2. Contusion	b.___ Puncture through the skin
3. Hematoma	c.___ Wound with break to the skin
4. Laceration	d.___ Wound with no break to the skin
5. Avulsion	e.___ Collection of blood under the tissues
6. Amputation	f.___ Scraping wound of the skin
7. Crush wound	g.___ Bruise
8. Open wound	h.___ Loose flap of skin
9. Closed wound	i.___ Loss of a body part or tissue
10. Penetration	j.___ Wound resulting from force applied to tissue

Section 12 – Soft Tissue Injuries

Review Questions – Multiple Choice

1. The nerve endings are found in which layer of the skin?

    a. Epidermis   b. Dermis   c. Subcutaneous tissue   d. Fascia

2. Open wounds are dangerous because of the potential for _____.

    a. Contamination   b. Scarring   c. Epithelialization   d. Granulation

3. A patient with a puncture wound in the soft tissues may also have suffered _____ _____ to underlying organs.

    a. Blunt trauma   b. Penetrating trauma   c. Closed trauma   d. Contusion trauma

4. Body Substance Isolation (BSI) considerations are important when preparing to care for a wounded individual.

    a. True   b. False

5. BSI considerations are only important to the diver medic and not the patient.

    a. True   b. False

6. Complete amputation of an extremity would warrant immediate application of a _____.

    a. Tourniquet   b. Occlusive dressing   c. Hemostatic agent   d. None of the above

7. Blast injuries result from all of the following, except;

    a. Primary phase   b. Secondary phase   c. Tertiary phase   d. Mechanism of injury

8. Which organs will suffer more severe injury during the 'primary' phase of a blast?

    a. Air filled   b. Solid   c. Voluntary   d. Liquid filled

9. During the 'secondary' phase of a blast event, most injuries are caused by _____.

    a. Flames   b. Pressure   c. Flying debris   d. Falling beams

10. Hemorrhage is generally classified as;

    a. Arterial / venous   b. Open / closed   c. Capillary   d. Spurting

11. Arterial bleeds are typically _____ and the blood will appear _____.

    a. Oozing / dull   b. Steady / bright   c. Spurting / bright   d. Steady / dull

12. Open, bleeding wounds are best treated initially with _____.

    a. Hemostats   b. Hemostatic agents   c. Tourniquet   d. Direct pressure

13. Venous bleeds are typically _____ and the blood will appear _____.

    a. Oozing / dull   b. Steady / bright   c. Spurting / bright   d. Steady / dull

Section 12 – Soft Tissue Injuries

14. A tourniquet should be applied how tight?

    a. Should never be applied   b. As tight as possible

    c. Tightened until the arterial bleed stops   d. Tighten until the venous bleed stops

15. Hemostatic agents are used to control _____ _____.

    a. All bleeding   b. Venous bleeds   c. Severe bleeding   d. Controlled bleeding

16. When applying hemostatic agents to a wound, the diver medic must still provide _____ _____ to the wound.

    a. Tourniquet   b. Direct pressure   c. Cold packs   d. Hemostats

17. Small wounds do not require cleaning.

    a. True   b. False

18. During this phase of healing, leucocytes (white blood cells) migrate to the wound site.

    a. Inflammation   b. Granulation   c. Epithelialization   d. Synthesis

19. Primary closure of a clean wound with little tissue loos should be performed within _____ hours.

    a. 12   b. 4 - 12   c. 6 - 8   d. 24

20. Direct infiltration requires injection of the anesthetic into the wound.

    a. True   b. False

21. Povidine-iodine (Betadine) should be diluted to a concentration of ____ % for cleaning internal wound areas.

    a. 4%   b. 6%   c. 10%   d. 1%

22. Placing sutures or staples closer together reduces wound tension.

    a. True   b. False

23. For deep tissue suturing, what type of sutures should be used?

    a. Vicryl   b. Nylon   c. Monofilament   d. Absorbable

24. 'Dead spaces', or 'pockets', in a sutured wound will increase the risk of _____.

    a. Healing   b. Scarring   c. Infection   d. None of the above

25. The 'Rule of Nines' is used to determine the total body surface area of a burn victim.

    a. True   b. False

26. The first step in caring for a burn victim is _____.

    a. Stop the burning   b. Apply wet dressings

    c. Apply dry dressings   d. Remove jewelry

Section 12 – Soft Tissue Injuries

27. First degree (superficial) burns may be treated using _____ dressings.

    a. Wet   b. Dry   c. Occlusive   d. Foil

28. Second degree (partial thickness) and third degree (full thickness) burns should be treated using a _____ dressing.

    a. Wet   b. Dry   c. Occlusive   d. Foil

29. Burn victims are at greater risk of _____ and _____.

    a. Infection / hyperthermia   b. Hypovolemia / hyperthermia

    c. Shock / hyperthermia   d. Infection / hypothermia

30. In reference to burn injuries, the 'Parkland Formula' is used to determine;

    a. Fluid requirements   b. Caloric requirements

    c. Pain management   d. Surface are burned

Label the correct 'Rule of Nines' percentages below

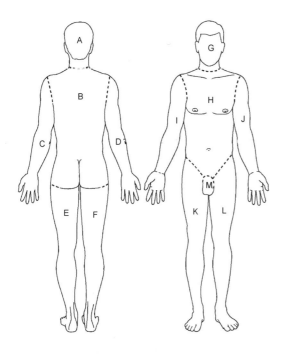

A._____
B._____
C._____
D._____
E._____
F._____
G._____
H._____
I._____
J._____
K._____
L._____
M._____

Section 12 – Soft Tissue Injuries

Find the Terms

A	B	R	A	S	I	O	N	D	G	Y	V	J	E	H
M	R	B	V	G	N	B	L	E	E	D	I	N	G	E
P	U	S	U	R	C	L	O	S	E	D	E	Y	A	M
U	I	T	L	F	I	R	O	F	C	A	T	T	N	M
T	S	A	S	A	S	U	T	U	R	E	N	F	G	O
A	E	P	T	H	I	B	U	R	N	S	A	C	R	R
T	O	L	O	S	O	F	T	R	W	G	M	H	E	A
I	O	E	N	Y	N	T	D	R	E	S	S	I	N	G
O	P	S	Q	U	I	K	C	L	O	T	K	T	E	E
N	E	C	R	O	S	I	S	W	F	U	J	O	G	S
D	N	E	C	O	L	L	A	G	E	N	R	S	J	U
E	C	L	A	M	P	H	E	M	O	S	T	A	T	T
R	W	O	U	N	D	C	A	R	E	O	T	N	L	U
Q	O	X	Y	G	E	N	T	F	O	R	C	E	P	R
T	O	U	R	N	I	Q	U	R	T	O	R	R	U	E

Abrasion
Amputation
Necrosis
Open
Incision
Avulsion
Bleeding
Vietnam
Suture
Closed
Dressing
Soft
CAT

Tourniquet
Wound care
Gangrene
Hemostat
Clamp
Forcep
Suture
Collagen
Burns
Staples
Quik clot
Celox
Oxygen

13 Musculoskeletal Injury

Fill In the Blanks

Label the Skeletal Structures

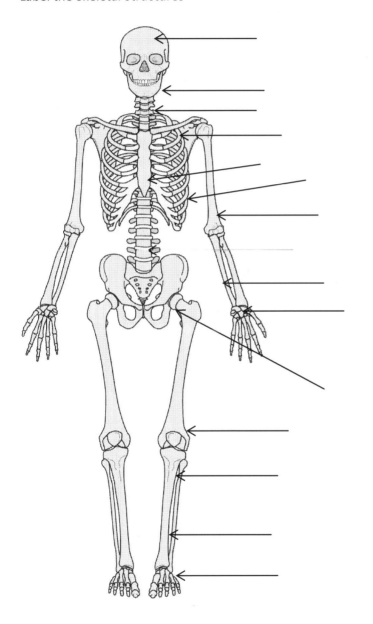

A. Patella

B. Femur

C. Ribs

D. Ulna

E. Radius

F. Tibia

G. Fibula

H. Skull

I. Humerus

J. Pelvis

K. Sternum

L. Clavicle

M. Mandible

N. Cervical vertebrae

O. Lumbar vertebrae

Section 13 – Musculoskeletal Injury

Mix and Match

Column 1   **Column 2**

1. _____ Angulation   a. Injury caused at the site of impact

2. _____ Direct Blow   b. Multiple fractures of the same bone with floating bone fragments

3. _____ Indirect Injury   c. Fracture caused by twisting motion

4. _____ Comminuted Fracture   d. A deformed fracture

5. _____ Greenstick Fracture   e. Fracture that has broken the skin

6. _____ Mechanism of Injury   f. Injury occurring remotely to the point of impact

7. _____ Closed Injury   g. Compression of bone ends together

8. _____ Open Injury   h. What events caused the injury

9. _____ Impacted Facture   i. Fracture that does not break the skin

10. _____ Spiral Fracture   j. Partial fracture of a bone

Label the Fractures

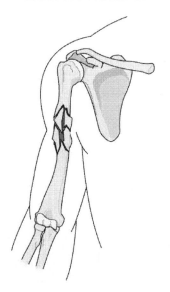 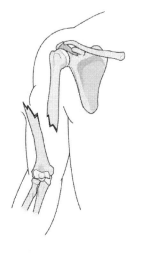 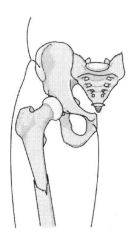

A. _____   B. _____   C. _____

Section 13 – Musculoskeletal Injury

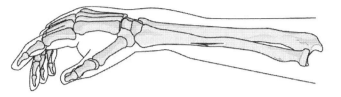 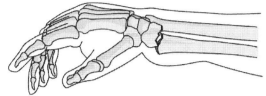

D._____   E._____

Review Questions – Multiple Choice

1. Muscles that we have no direct control over are called _____ or _____ muscles.

    a. Voluntary / cardiac   b. Skeletal / smooth

    c. Involuntary / smooth   d. Involuntary / skeletal

2. Skeletal muscles are attached to _____.

    a. Bones   b. Joints   c. Ligaments   d. Smooth muscles

3. The skeletal muscles are attached to the bones via _____.

    a. Ligaments   b. Tendons   c. Joints   d. Suture joints

4. Joints are stabilized by _____.

    a. Bones   b. Joints   c. Ligaments   d. Smooth muscles

5. The inner portion of the bone is known as the _____ and produces red blood cells.

    a. Condyle   b. Marrow   c. Tuberosity   d. Iliac

6. _____, _____, and _____ must be evaluated before and after splinting.

    a. Circulation, motor, sensory   b. Color, temperature, appearance

    c. Circulation, temperature, pulse   d. Pulse, movement, color

7. Traction splints should be used for fractures:

    a. At or near mid-femur   b. Of the lower leg

    c. Only on closed factures   d. Only on open fractures

67

Section 13 – Musculoskeletal Injury

8. The joints above and below a joint injury should be immobilized.

    a. True   b. False

9. The joints above and below a bone injury should be immobilized

    a. True   b. False

10. A disruption of a joint in which the bone ends are no longer in contact is called a _____.

    a. Sprain   b. Fracture   c. Strain   d. Dislocation

11. A strain is classified as an injury to the _____.

    a. Bones   b. Tendons   c. Ligaments   d. Muscles

12. A sprain is classified as an injury to the _____.

    a. Bones   b. Tendons   c. Ligaments   d. Muscles

13. Reliable signs and symptoms of a fracture include all of these except:

    a. Point tenderness   b. Pain   c. Deformity   d. Cyanosis

14. Point tenderness is considered the most reliable indicator of a bone injury.

    a. True   b. False

15. Dislocations can damage _____ and _____ if not treated appropriately.

    a. Muscles / tendons   b. Blood vessels / nerves

    c. Ligaments / Joints   d. Muscles / bones

16. 95% of shoulder dislocations are _____ dislocations.

    a. Anterior   b. Posterior   c. Proximal   d. Distal

17. Loss of a _____ _____ in an injured limb could indicate that the blood vessels are compromised.

    a. Proximal pulse   b. Distal pulse   c. Dorsal   d. Ventral

18. The elbow is considered a _____ joint.

    a. Rolling   b. Ball and socket   c. Hinged   d. Rotating

19. The most commonly injured joint is the _____.

    a. Hip   b. Knee   c. Elbow   d. Ankle

20. A grating or grinding noise at the site of a bone injury is known as _____.

    a. Fowlers response   b. Point tenderness   c. Rales   d. Crepitus

14 Cardiac Emergencies

Mix and Match

Match the terms in the first column with the definitions in the second column.

1. _____ Left ventricle	a. Thick wall of muscle separating the chambers

2. _____ Aorta	b. Provides electronic delay following atrial depolarization

3. _____ Right ventricle	c. Pumps oxygenated blood into the system

4. _____ Sinus Atrial Node	d. Receives deoxygenated blood from the system

5. _____ Purkinje Network	e. Pumps deoxygenated blood to the lungs

6. _____ Right Atrium	f. Receives oxygenated blood from the lungs

7. _____ Septum	g. Primary electrical pacemaker

8. _____ Left Atrium	h. Network of electrical fibers surrounding the ventricles

9. _____ Bundle of HIS	i. Secondary pacemaker if the primary fails

10. _____ AV Node	j. Largest artery in the body

Review Questions – Multiple Choice

1. Current American Heart Association standards call for a circulation check first, in the initial assessment.

    a. True	b. False

2. A pulse check on a victim should last no more than how many seconds?

    a. 15	b. 20	c. 10	d. 25

3. To open the airway of a non-spinal injured victim, we use which technique?

    a. Head tilt / chin lift	b. Jaw thrust	c. Finger sweep	d. Head tilt / neck lift

4. The recommended minimum depth of compression in inches on an adult victim is;

    a. 1	b. 2	c. 2.5	d. 3

5. The compression / ventilation ratio for single rescuer CPR is what?

    a. 15:1	b. 5:1	c. 30:2	d. 15:2

6. What is the recommended rate of compressions for all victims?

    a. 60-80 per minute	b. 80-99 per minute	c. 100-120 per minute	d. 40 per minute

Section 14 – Cardiac Emergencies

7. To avoid gastric distention when using a bag valve mask, it is recommended that you;

    a. Give a breath until you see the chest rise   b. Give long, slow breaths

    c. Give breaths quickly   d. Give the most breaths you can

8. Adequate depth of compressions is needed during CPR to;

    a. Prolong ventricular fibrillation   b. Create blood flow

    c. Create airflow   d. None of the above

9. When using an Automated External Defibrillator (AED), the first set is to;

    a. Turn the unit on   b. Attach the pads   c. Connect the pads   d. None of the above

10. During 2 rescuer CPR, the first rescuer maintains airway and breathing, what does the second rescuer do?

    a. Calls for help   b. Provides chest compressions

    c. Inserts an advanced airway   d. Checks the victim's pulse

11. After the AED delivers a shock, you should;

    a. Immediately begin chest compressions   b. Wait for the AED to reanalyze the victim

    c. Insert an advanced airway   d. Pulse check

12. With regards to chest compressions, the rescuer should place their hands where;

    a. Abdomen   b. Lower half of the sternum

    b. Upper half of the sternum   d. Middle of the sternum

13. A rescuers first action for a victim of a foreign body airway obstruction is to;

    a. Provide abdominal thrusts   b. Chest thrusts

    c. Blind finger sweep   d. CPR

14. Compression / ventilation rates with 2 rescuers and an advanced airway in place is;

    a. 100 / 6-8   b. 120 / 5-10   c. 100 / 5-10   d. 120 / 6-8

15. When should you move an adult victim who requires CPR?

    a. After 15 minutes of CPR   b. As soon as you have enough resources

    c. When the scene is unsafe   d. Never move the victim

15 – Related Medical Procedures

Review Questions – Multiple Choice

1. Foley catheterization is a skill utilized when an injured diver presents and cannot _____.

    a. Breath   b. Urinate   c. Defecate   d. Swallow

2. The cuff at the end of a Foley catheter is filled with _____ once the catheter has been inserted.

    a. Water   b. Sterile water   c. Normal saline   d. All of the above

3. Air cannot be used to fill the cuff of the catheter due to what gas law?

    a. Boyle's Law   b. Dalton's Law   c. Henry's Law   d. Charles Law

4. The Foley is inserted into the _____ via the _____.

    a. Kidneys / urethra   b. Bladder / ureter   c. Bladder / urethra   d. Kidneys / ureter

5. In a male patient, the Foley must pass through what gland prior to entering the bladder?

    a. Urethra   b. Ureter   c. Meatus   d. Prostate

6. A needle thoracentesis is a procedure that may need to be performed on a diver with thoracic trauma?

    a. True   b. False

7. A 2-inch 14-gauge catheter is acceptable to decompress the chest of an injured diver.

    a. True   b. False

8. What length and gauge of catheter should be used to decompress the chest of an injured diver?

    a. 2 inch / 16 gauge   b. 2 inch / 14 gauge   c. 3 inch / 12 gauge   d. 3 inch / 16 gauge

9. A pneumothorax is an immediate life-threatening injury.

    a. True   b. False

10. A simple pneumothorax can develop into a _____ pneumothorax if air continues to leak from the injured lung.

    a. Spontaneous   b. Tension   c. Simple   d. Complex

11. A late sign of a tension pneumothorax is tracheal deviation to the _____.

    a. Left   b. Right   c. Affected side   d. Unaffected side

Section 15 – Related Medical Procedures

12. The _____ intercostal space on the affected side is the preferred insertion point for the catheter when decompressing the chest of an injured diver.

    a. 2nd   b. 3rd   c. 4th   d. It does not matter

13. When addressing open chest trauma, the diver medic should initially seal the wound in the chest.

    a. True   b. False

14. If an occlusive dressing is applied to an open chest wound, the diver medic must monitor the patient for the development of a _____.

    a. Tension pneumothorax   b. Simple pneumothorax

    c. Cardiac arrhythmia   d. Shortness of breath

15. After applying an occlusive dressing to an open chest wound, if a tension pneumothorax develops, the diver medic should _____.

    a. Leave the dressing in place   b. Completely remove the dressing

    c. Lift one corner of the dressing to release air   d. Tell the patient to stop whining

16. An inserted chest tube must be connected to a(n) _____ to avoid having air drawn back into the chest cavity.

    a. Water seal   b. Heimlich valve   c. Asherman seal   d. Vacuum seal

17. Inserting a chest tube is a surgical procedure.

    a. True   b. False

18. The correct insertion point for a chest tube is the _____ intercostal space.

    a. 1st or 2nd   b. 3rd or 4th   c. 4th or 5th   d. Below the nipple line

19. The Asherman chest seal allows air to escape the thoracic cavity if pressure builds.

    a. True   b. False

20. A hemothorax is defined as an accumulation of _____ in the thoracic cavity.

    a. Gas   b. Air   c. Blood   d. Fluid

Section 16 – Saturation Diving Issues

Review Questions – Multiple Choice

1. An injured diver in saturation poses a special problem for the diver medic because;

    a. They cannot 'lockout' for treatment   b. They need to be 'surfaced' for treatment

    c. The habitat is too small   d. The habitat contains a heliox breathing mix

2. Diving Medical Officers (DMO) routinely 'lock-in' to assist diver medics in the treatment of injured divers.

    a. True   b. False

3. The Diving Medical Advisory Committee (DMAC), routinely issues advisories to assist the diver medic with direction on care and treatment of injured and ill divers in saturation.

    a. True   b. False

4. The diver medic will most likely be in-charge of the medical supplies and equipment held on site or in the diving bell. How often should the diver medic inspect and log that inspection of these supplies?

    a. 1 – 2 months   b. 3 – 6 months   c. Yearly   d. As needed

5. DMAC, NOAA, and the US Navy all have requirements for medical equipment to be held on site of diving operations.

    a. True   b. False

6. A diver medic working in saturation will be responsible for designating a work area in the event of a medical emergency.

    a. True   b. False

7. If working from a bell during a medical emergency, the first challenge for the diver medic is _____ the injured diver.

    a. Communicating with   b. Locating   c. Retrieving   d. Removing dive gear from

8. In a life-threatening emergency, the removed dive gear; i.e. helmet and umbilicals, the diver medic may need to _____ this gear _____.

    a. Stow / in the bell locker   b. Dump / overboard

    c. Stow / on the bottom of the bell   d. None of the above

9. A major issue for the diver medic working in the bell during a medical emergency is _____.

    a. The helium environment   b. The lack of available space

    c. The bilging of the bell   d. Limited supplies of breathing gas

Section 16 – Saturation Diving Issues

10. Patient transfer from the bell to the designated treatment area inside the saturation habitat can be accomplished using rope or web slings, and / or a commercial canvas stretcher.

    a. True   b. False

11. Lost bell incidents are rare; however, the major issue affecting the bell divers will be _____.

    a. Hypothermia   b. Dehydration   c. Hyperthermia   d. Claustrophobia

12. With proper emergency equipment; i.e. survival suit and CO_2 scrubbers, survival times can reach up to _____ hours for the diver inside of a lost bell.

    a. 36   b. 12   c. 48   d. 24

13. Hyperbaric lifeboats contain a habitat chamber pressurized to the same depth as the saturation habitat.

    a. True   b. False

14. A Hyperbaric Rescue Chamber (HRC) is lowered into the water and makes way under its own power.

    a. True   b. False

15. Emergency locator transmitters are required on all hyperbaric lifeboats and rescue chambers.

    a. True   b. False

17 Live Bait

Review Questions – Multiple Choice

1. In many cases, the only means to evacuate an injured diver will be by _____ or _____.

    a. Land / water   b. Water / air   c. Land / air   d. TUP / land

2. As a diver medic transporting an injured diver, the first responsibility of the diver medic is to insure that the injured diver is _____.

    a. Hydrated   b. Warm   c. Fed   d. Protected

3. If transporting an injured diver in a boat in rough seas, the boat should be moving _____.

    a. To starboard   b. Slowly   c. Quickly   d. None of these

4. If transporting an injured diver in a non-pressurized aircraft, the altitude of that aircraft should not exceed _____ feet above ground level.

    a. 500   b. 1,000   c. 10,000   d. 2,000

5. In a pressurized aircraft, the cabin pressure should be maintain as close as possible to _____.

    a. 14.7 psi / 760 mmHg   b. 29.4 psi / 1520 mmHg

    c. 1 ATA   d. Both a. and c.

6. In a modern airliner, a cabin pressure of 1 ATA can be achieved by descending to an altitude of _____.

    a. 18,000 – 21,000 feet MSL   b. 10,000 – 15,000 feet MSL

    c. 10,000 – 12,000 feet AGL   d. It is not possible to pressurize to 1 ATA

7. Approaching a rescue helicopter from the rear is an acceptable practice for the diver medic.

    a. True   b. False

8. Helicopters have absolutely no need to take-off and land into the wind.

    a. True   b. False

9. The accepted touchdown, (landing areas), areas for helicopters during the day is _____ by _____.

    a. 60 feet ,18 meters / 60 feet, 18 meters   b. 75 feet, 23 meters / 75 feet, 23 meters

    c. 120 feet, 36 meters / 120 feet, 36 meters   d. Any area with loose debris

10. The accepted touchdown area for a helicopter during the night is _____ by _____.

    a. 60 feet ,18 meters / 60 feet, 18 meters   b. 75 feet, 23 meters / 75 feet, 23 meters

    c. 100 feet, 33 meters / 100 feet, 33 meters   d. Any area with loose debris

Section 17 – Live Bait

11. The four corners of a helicopter landing zone should be marked with something that will be visible to the pilot.

    a. True   b. False

12. The use of flares is encouraged by many EMS helicopter pilots.

    a. True   b. False

13. During night operations with EMS helicopters, it is recommended that flashlights be directed at, and waved at the inbound aircraft is insure that the landing site is located by the pilot.

    a. True   b. False

14. Shining lights at the helicopter crew during night operations will compromise their _____.

    a. Night vision   b. Coordination   c. Aircraft   d. None of these

15. The diver medic should never approach the helicopter unless directed to do so by the crew.

    a. True   b. False

16. In rear loading helicopters, the _____ is the most serious hazard.

    a. Debris   b. Rotor wash   c. Lighting   d. Tail rotor

17. A 'hot' load of a helicopter means that the aircraft is _____ during loading of the patient.

    a. Shutdown   b. Left running   c. Secured   d. None of these

18. Once the helicopter departs the landing zone, the site should be kept secure for at least _____ minutes.

    a. 5   b. 15   c. 30   d. 60

19. A chamber tender or diver medic will not be allowed to fly for _____ hours after completing US Navy Treatment Tables 5, 6, 6A.

    a. 72   b. 36   c. 24   d. 12

20. A civilian diver receiving hyperbaric treatments for a diving injury should not be allowed to fly for at least _____ to _____ days.

    a. 3 / 5   b. 1 / 2   c. 2 / 3   d. 5 / 7

21. Female divers normally have lower oxygen demands than their male counterparts do.

    a. True   b. False

22. A pregnant female diver will not put the fetus at risk if diving shallow.

    a. True   b. False

23. Oxygen is a flammable, explosive gas.

    a. True   b. False

24. Brass oxygen regulators will not burn in a pure oxygen environment because brass is a non-ferrous metal.

    a. True   b. False

25. Quarter turn valves are safe to install on all oxygen system lines.

    a. True   b. False

26. Which valve is acceptable for installation on a pressurized oxygen system?

    a. Quarter turn valve   b. Needle metering valve   c. Ball valve   d. Plate valve

27. Regulators attached to portable oxygen tanks utilize a special configuration to attach to the valve stem known as _____.

    a. Pin indexing system   b. Color coding system

    c. Bourdon attachment system   d. None of these

28. All compressed gas tanks follow the same marking identifiers worldwide.

    a. True   b. False

29. Large oxygen tanks are normally equipped with a CGA _____ fitting.

    a. 870   b. 747   c. 540   d. XYZ

30. A pressure reduction regulator is used to regulate the oxygen pressure being sent to an oxygen delivery device such as a BIBS.

    a. True   b. False

Appendix

Use these Tables for Calculations

Depth (fsw)	No-Stop Limit	Repetitive Group Designation															
		A	B	C	D	E	F	G	H	I	J	K	L	M	N	O	Z
10	Unlimited	57	101	158	245	426	*										
15	Unlimited	36	60	88	121	163	217	297	449	*							
20	Unlimited	26	43	61	82	106	133	165	205	256	330	461	*				
25	595	20	33	47	62	78	97	117	140	166	198	236	285	354	469	595	
30	371	17	27	38	50	62	76	91	107	125	145	167	193	223	260	307	371
35	232	14	23	32	42	52	63	74	87	100	115	131	148	168	190	215	232
40	163	12	20	27	36	44	53	63	73	84	95	108	121	135	151	163	
45	125	11	17	24	31	39	46	55	63	72	82	92	102	114	125		
50	92	9	15	21	28	34	41	48	56	63	71	80	89	92			
55	74	8	14	19	25	31	37	43	50	56	63	71	74				
60	60	7	12	17	22	28	33	39	45	51	57	60					
70	48	6	10	14	19	23	28	32	37	42	47	48					
80	39	5	9	12	16	20	24	28	32	36	39						
90	30	4	7	11	14	17	21	24	28	30							
100	25	4	6	9	12	15	18	21	25								
110	20	3	6	8	11	14	16	19	20								
120	15	3	5	7	10	12	15										
130	10	2	4	6	9	10											
140	10	2	4	6	8	10											
150	5	2	3	5													
160	5		3	5													
170	5			4	5												
180	5			4	5												
190	5			3	5												

* Highest repetitive group that can be achieved at this depth regardless of bottom time.

U.S. Navy No-Deco Table

Appendix

Table 9-8. Residual Nitrogen Time Table for Repetitive Air Dives.

Locate the diver's repetitive group designation from his previous dive along the diagonal line above the table. Read horizontally to the interval in which the diver's surface interval lies.

Next, read vertically downward to the new repetitive group designation. Continue downward in this same column to the row that represents the depth of the repetitive dive. The time given at the intersection is residual nitrogen time, in minutes, to be applied to the repetitive dive.

* Dives following surface intervals longer than this are not repetitive dives. Use actual bottom times in the Air Decompression Tables to compute decompression for such dives.

Repetitive Group at Beginning of Surface Interval

Group															
A														:10	2:20 *
B													:10	1:17	
												1:16	3:36 *		
C												:10	:56	2:12	
											:55	2:11	4:31 *		
D											:10	:53	1:48	3:04	
										:52	1:47	3:03	5:23 *		
E										:10	:53	1:45	2:40	3:56	
									:52	1:44	2:39	3:55	6:15 *		
F									:10	:53	1:45	2:38	3:32	4:49	
								:52	1:44	2:37	3:31	4:48	7:08 *		
G								:10	:53	1:45	2:38	3:30	4:24	5:41	
							:52	1:44	2:37	3:29	4:23	5:40	8:00 *		
H							:10	:53	1:45	2:38	3:30	4:22	5:17	6:33	
						:52	1:44	2:37	3:29	4:21	5:16	6:32	8:52 *		
I						:10	:53	1:45	2:38	3:30	4:22	5:14	6:09	7:25	
					:52	1:44	2:37	3:29	4:21	5:13	6:08	7:24	9:44 *		
J					:10	:53	1:45	2:38	3:30	4:22	5:14	6:07	7:01	8:17	
					:52	1:44	2:37	3:29	4:21	5:13	6:06	7:00	8:16	10:36 *	
K				:10	:53	1:45	2:38	3:30	4:22	5:14	6:07	6:59	7:53	9:10	
				:52	1:44	2:37	3:29	4:21	5:13	6:06	6:58	7:52	9:09	11:29 *	
L			:10	:53	1:45	2:38	3:30	4:22	5:14	6:07	6:59	7:51	8:45	10:02	
			:52	1:44	2:37	3:29	4:21	5:13	6:06	6:58	7:50	8:44	10:01	12:21 *	
M		:10	:53	1:45	2:38	3:30	4:22	5:14	6:07	6:59	7:51	8:43	9:38	10:54	
		:52	1:44	2:37	3:29	4:21	5:13	6:06	6:58	7:50	8:42	9:37	10:53	13:13 *	
N	:10	:53	1:45	2:38	3:30	4:22	5:14	6:07	6:59	7:51	8:43	9:35	10:30	11:46	
	:52	1:44	2:37	3:29	4:21	5:13	6:06	6:58	7:50	8:42	9:34	10:29	11:45	14:05 *	
O	:10	:53	1:45	2:38	3:30	4:22	5:14	6:07	6:59	7:51	8:43	9:35	10:28	11:22	12:38
	:52	1:44	2:37	3:29	4:21	5:13	6:06	6:58	7:50	8:42	9:34	10:27	11:21	12:37	14:58 *
Z	:10	:53	1:45	2:38	3:30	4:22	5:14	6:07	6:59	7:51	8:43	9:35	10:28	11:20	12:14	13:31
	:52	1:44	2:37	3:29	4:21	5:13	6:06	6:58	7:50	8:42	9:34	10:27	11:19	12:13	13:30	15:50 *

Repetitive Group at the End of the Surface Interval

Dive Depth	Z	O	N	M	L	K	J	I	H	G	F	E	D	C	B	A
10	**	**	**	**	**	**	**	**	**	**	**	427	246	159	101	58
15	**	**	**	**	**	**	**	**	450	298	218	164	122	89	61	37
20	**	**	**	**	**	462	331	257	206	166	134	106	83	62	44	27
25	†	†	470	354	286	237	198	167	141	118	98	79	63	48	34	21
30	372	308	261	224	194	168	146	126	108	92	77	63	51	39	28	18
35	245	216	191	169	149	132	116	101	88	75	64	53	43	33	24	15
40	188	169	152	136	122	109	97	85	74	64	55	45	37	29	21	13
45	154	140	127	115	104	93	83	73	64	56	48	40	32	25	18	12
50	131	120	109	99	90	81	73	65	57	49	42	35	29	23	17	11
55	114	105	96	88	80	72	65	58	51	44	38	32	26	20	15	10
60	101	93	86	79	72	65	58	52	46	40	35	29	24	19	14	9
70	83	77	71	65	59	54	49	44	39	34	29	25	20	16	12	8
80	70	65	60	55	51	46	42	38	33	29	25	22	18	14	10	7
90	61	57	52	48	44	41	37	33	29	26	22	19	16	12	9	6
100	54	50	47	43	40	36	33	30	26	23	20	17	14	11	8	5
110	48	45	42	39	36	33	30	27	24	21	18	16	13	10	8	5
120	44	41	38	35	32	30	27	24	22	19	17	14	12	9	7	5
130	40	37	35	32	30	27	25	22	20	18	15	13	11	9	6	4
140	37	34	32	30	27	25	23	21	19	16	14	12	10	8	6	4
150	34	32	30	28	26	23	21	19	17	15	13	11	9	8	6	4
160	32	30	28	26	24	22	20	18	16	14	13	11	9	7	5	4
170	30	28	26	24	22	21	19	17	15	14	12	10	8	7	5	3
180	28	26	25	23	21	19	18	16	14	13	11	10	8	6	5	3
190	26	25	23	22	20	18	17	15	14	12	11	9	8	6	5	3

Residual Nitrogen Times (Minutes)

** Residual Nitrogen Time cannot be determined using this table (see paragraph 9-9.1 subparagraph 8 for instructions).
† Read vertically downward to the 30 fsw repetitive dive depth. Use the corresponding residual nitrogen times to compute the equivalent single dive time. Decompress using the 30 fsw air decompression table.

U.S. Navy Residual Nitrogen Table

Appendix

US Navy Air / Oxygen Decompression Tables

(DESCENT RATE 75 FPM—ASCENT RATE 30 FPM)

Bottom Time (min)	Time to First Stop (M:S)	Gas Mix	Decompression Stops (FSW) Stop times (min) include travel time, except first air and first O₂ stop									Total Ascent Time (M:S)	Chamber O₂ Periods	Repet Group
			100	90	80	70	60	50	40	30	20			
30 FSW														
371	1:00	AIR									0	1:00	0	Z
		AIR/O₂									0	1:00		
380	0:20	AIR									5	6:00	0.5	Z
		AIR/O₂									1	2:00		
In-Water Air/O₂ Decompression or SurDO₂ Recommended														
420	0:20	AIR									22	23:00	0.5	Z
		AIR/O₂									5	6:00		
480	0:20	AIR									42	43:00	0.5	
		AIR/O₂									9	10:00		
540	0:20	AIR									71	72:00	1	
		AIR/O₂									14	15:00		
Exceptional Exposure: In-Water Air Decompression ———— In-Water Air/O₂ Decompression or SurDO₂ Required														
600	0:20	AIR									92	93:00	1	
		AIR/O₂									19	20:00		
660	0:20	AIR									120	121:00	1	
		AIR/O₂									22	23:00		
720	0:20	AIR									158	159:00	1	
		AIR/O₂									27	28:00		
35 FSW														
232	1:10	AIR									0	1:10	0	Z
		AIR/O₂									0	1:10		
240	0:30	AIR									4	5:10	0.5	Z
		AIR/O₂									2	3:10		
In-Water Air/O₂ Decompression or SurDO₂ Recommended														
270	0:30	AIR									28	29:10	0.5	Z
		AIR/O₂									7	8:10		
300	0:30	AIR									53	54:10	0.5	Z
		AIR/O₂									13	14:10		
330	0:30	AIR									71	72:10	1	Z
		AIR/O₂									18	19:10		
360	0:30	AIR									88	89:10	1	
		AIR/O₂									22	23:10		
Exceptional Exposure: In-Water Air Decompression ———— In-Water Air/O₂ Decompression or SurDO₂ Required														
420	0:30	AIR									134	135:10	1.5	
		AIR/O₂									29	30:10		
480	0:30	AIR									173	174:10	1.5	
		AIR/O₂									38	44:10		
540	0:30	AIR									228	229:10	2	
		AIR/O₂									45	51:10		
600	0:30	AIR									277	278:10	2	
		AIR/O₂									53	59:10		
660	0:30	AIR									314	315:10	2.5	
		AIR/O₂									63	69:10		
720	0:30	AIR									342	343:10	3	
		AIR/O₂									71	82:10		

Appendix

(DESCENT RATE 75 FPM—ASCENT RATE 30 FPM)

Bottom Time (min)	Time to First Stop (M:S)	Gas Mix	Decompression Stops (FSW) Stop times (min) include travel time, except first air and first O₂ stop									Total Ascent Time (M:S)	Chamber O₂ Periods	Repet Group
			100	90	80	70	60	50	40	30	20			
40 FSW														
163	1:20	AIR									0	1:20	0	O
		AIR/O₂									0	1:20		
170	0:40	AIR									6	7:20	0.5	O
		AIR/O₂									2	3:20		
180	0:40	AIR									14	15:20	0.5	Z
		AIR/O₂									5	6:20		
In-Water Air/O₂ Decompression or SurDO₂ Recommended														
190	0:40	AIR									21	22:20	0.5	Z
		AIR/O₂									7	8:20		
200	0:40	AIR									27	28:20	0.5	Z
		AIR/O₂									9	10:20		
210	0:40	AIR									39	40:20	0.5	Z
		AIR/O₂									11	12:20		
220	0:40	AIR									52	53:20	0.5	Z
		AIR/O₂									12	13:20		
230	0:40	AIR									64	65:20	1	Z
		AIR/O₂									16	17:20		
240	0:40	AIR									75	76:20	1	Z
		AIR/O₂									19	20:20		
Exceptional Exposure: In-Water Air Decompression ------------ In-Water Air/O₂ Decompression or SurDO₂ Required -----------														
270	0:40	AIR									101	102:20	1	Z
		AIR/O₂									26	27:20		
300	0:40	AIR									128	129:20	1.5	
		AIR/O₂									33	34:20		
330	0:40	AIR									160	161:20	1.5	
		AIR/O₂									38	44:20		
360	0:40	AIR									184	185:20	2	
		AIR/O₂									44	50:20		
420	0:40	AIR									248	249:20	2.5	
		AIR/O₂									56	62:20		
480	0:40	AIR									321	322:20	2.5	
		AIR/O₂									68	79:20		
Exceptional Exposure: In-Water Air/O₂ Decompression ------------ SurDO₂ Required--------------------------------------														
540	0:40	AIR									372	373:20	3	
		AIR/O₂									80	91:20		
600	0:40	AIR									410	411:20	3.5	
		AIR/O₂									93	104:20		
660	0:40	AIR									439	440:20	4	
		AIR/O₂									103	119:20		
Exceptional Exposure: SurDO₂ --														
720	0:40	AIR									461	462:20	4.5	
		AIR/O₂									112	128:20		

Appendix

(DESCENT RATE 75 FPM—ASCENT RATE 30 FPM)

Bottom Time (min)	Time to First Stop (M:S)	Gas Mix	DECOMPRESSION STOPS (FSW) Stop times (min) include travel time, except first air and first O₂ stop									Total Ascent Time (M:S)	Chamber O₂ Periods	Repet Group
			100	90	80	70	60	50	40	30	20			

45 FSW

Bottom Time (min)	Time to First Stop (M:S)	Gas Mix	100	90	80	70	60	50	40	30	20	Total Ascent Time (M:S)	Chamber O₂ Periods	Repet Group
125	1:30	AIR									0	1:30	0	N
		AIR/O₂									0	1:30		
130	0:50	AIR									2	3:30	0.5	O
		AIR/O₂									1	2:30		
140	0:50	AIR									14	15:30	0.5	O
		AIR/O₂									5	6:30		
In-Water Air/O₂ Decompression or SurDO₂ Recommended														
150	0:50	AIR									25	26:30	0.5	Z
		AIR/O₂									8	9:30		
160	0:50	AIR									34	35:30	0.5	Z
		AIR/O₂									11	12:30		
170	0:50	AIR									41	42:30	1	Z
		AIR/O₂									14	15:30		
180	0:50	AIR									59	60:30	1	Z
		AIR/O₂									17	18:30		
190	0:50	AIR									75	76:30	1	Z
		AIR/O₂									19	20:30		
Exceptional Exposure: In-Water Air Decompression ----- In-Water Air/O₂ Decompression or SurDO₂ Required -----														
200	0:50	AIR									89	90:30	1	Z
		AIR/O₂									23	24:30		
210	0:50	AIR									101	102:30	1	Z
		AIR/O₂									27	28:30		
220	0:50	AIR									112	113:30	1.5	Z
		AIR/O₂									30	31:30		
230	0:50	AIR									121	122:30	1.5	Z
		AIR/O₂									33	34:30		
240	0:50	AIR									130	131:30	1.5	Z
		AIR/O₂									37	43:30		
270	0:50	AIR									173	174:30	2	
		AIR/O₂									45	51:30		
300	0:50	AIR									206	207:30	2	
		AIR/O₂									51	57:30		
330	0:50	AIR									243	244:30	2.5	
		AIR/O₂									61	67:30		
360	0:50	AIR									288	289:30	3	
		AIR/O₂									69	80:30		
Exceptional Exposure: In-Water Air/O₂ Decompression ----- SurDO₂ Required -----														
420	0:50	AIR									373	374:30	3.5	
		AIR/O₂									84	95:30		
480	0:50	AIR									431	432:30	4	
		AIR/O₂									101	117:30		
Exceptional Exposure: SurDO₂ -----														
540	0:50	AIR									473	474:30	4.5	
		AIR/O₂									117	133:30		

Appendix

(DESCENT RATE 75 FPM—ASCENT RATE 30 FPM)

Bottom Time (min)	Time to First Stop (M:S)	Gas Mix	100	90	80	70	60	50	40	30	20	Total Ascent Time (M:S)	Chamber O_2 Periods	Repet Group
50 FSW														
92	1:40	AIR									0	1:40	0	M
		AIR/O_2									0	1:40		
95	1:00	AIR									2	3:40	0.5	M
		AIR/O_2									1	2:40		
100	1:00	AIR									4	5:40	0.5	N
		AIR/O_2									2	3:40		
110	1:00	AIR									8	9:40	0.5	O
		AIR/O_2									4	5:40		
In-Water Air/O_2 Decompression or SurDO_2 Recommended														
120	1:00	AIR									21	22:40	0.5	O
		AIR/O_2									7	8:40		
130	1:00	AIR									34	35:40	0.5	Z
		AIR/O_2									12	13:40		
140	1:00	AIR									45	46:40	1	Z
		AIR/O_2									16	17:40		
150	1:00	AIR									56	57:40	1	Z
		AIR/O_2									19	20:40		
160	1:00	AIR									78	79:40	1	Z
		AIR/O_2									23	24:40		
Exceptional Exposure: In-Water Air Decompression ———— In-Water Air/O_2 Decompression or SurDO_2 Required														
170	1:00	AIR									96	97:40	1	Z
		AIR/O_2									26	27:40		
180	1:00	AIR									111	112:40	1.5	Z
		AIR/O_2									30	31:40		
190	1:00	AIR									125	126:40	1.5	Z
		AIR/O_2									35	36:40		
200	1:00	AIR									136	137:40	1.5	Z
		AIR/O_2									39	45:40		
210	1:00	AIR									147	148:40	2	
		AIR/O_2									43	49:40		
220	1:00	AIR									166	167:40	2	
		AIR/O_2									47	53:40		
230	1:00	AIR									183	184:40	2	
		AIR/O_2									50	56:40		
240	1:00	AIR									198	199:40	2	
		AIR/O_2									53	59:40		
270	1:00	AIR									236	237:40	2.5	
		AIR/O_2									62	68:40		
300	1:00	AIR									285	286:40	3	
		AIR/O_2									74	85:40		
Exceptional Exposure: In-Water Air/O_2 Decompression ———— SurDO_2 Required														
330	1:00	AIR									345	346:40	3.5	
		AIR/O_2									83	94:40		
360	1:00	AIR									393	394:40	3.5	
		AIR/O_2									92	103:40		
Exceptional Exposure: SurDO_2														
420	1:00	AIR									464	465:40	4.5	
		AIR/O_2									113	129:40		

Appendix

(DESCENT RATE 75 FPM—ASCENT RATE 30 FPM)

Bottom Time (min)	Time to First Stop (M:S)	Gas Mix	Decompression Stops (FSW) 100	90	80	70	60	50	40	30	20	Total Ascent Time (M:S)	Chamber O_2 Periods	Repet Group
55 FSW														
74	1:50	AIR									0	1:50	0	L
		AIR/O_2									0	1:50		
75	1:10	AIR									1	2:50	0.5	L
		AIR/O_2									1	2:50		
80	1:10	AIR									4	5:50	0.5	M
		AIR/O_2									2	3:50		
90	1:10	AIR									10	11:50	0.5	N
		AIR/O_2									5	6:50		
In-Water Air/O_2 Decompression or SurDO$_2$ Recommended ---														
100	1:10	AIR									17	18:50	0.5	O
		AIR/O_2									8	9:50		
110	1:10	AIR									34	35:50	0.5	O
		AIR/O_2									12	13:50		
120	1:10	AIR									48	49:50	1	Z
		AIR/O_2									17	18:50		
130	1:10	AIR									59	60:50	1	Z
		AIR/O_2									22	23:50		
140	1:10	AIR									84	85:50	1	Z
		AIR/O_2									26	27:50		
Exceptional Exposure: In-Water Air Decompression ------------ In-Water Air/O_2 Decompression or SurDO$_2$ Required ----------														
150	1:10	AIR									105	106:50	1.5	Z
		AIR/O_2									30	31:50		
160	1:10	AIR									123	124:50	1.5	Z
		AIR/O_2									34	35:50		
170	1:10	AIR									138	139:50	1.5	Z
		AIR/O_2									40	46:50		
180	1:10	AIR									151	152:50	2	Z
		AIR/O_2									45	51:50		
190	1:10	AIR									169	170:50	2	
		AIR/O_2									50	56:50		
200	1:10	AIR									190	191:50	2	
		AIR/O_2									54	60:50		
210	1:10	AIR									208	209:50	2.5	
		AIR/O_2									58	64:50		
220	1:10	AIR									224	225:50	2.5	
		AIR/O_2									62	68:50		
230	1:10	AIR									239	240:50	2.5	
		AIR/O_2									66	77:50		
240	1:10	AIR									254	255:50	3	
		AIR/O_2									69	80:50		
Exceptional Exposure: In-Water Air/O_2 Decompression ------------ SurDO$_2$ Required--------------------------------														
270	1:10	AIR									313	314:50	3.5	
		AIR/O_2									83	94:50		
300	1:10	AIR									380	381:50	3.5	
		AIR/O_2									94	105:50		
330	1:10	AIR									432	433:50	4	
		AIR/O_2									106	122:50		
Exceptional Exposure: SurDO$_2$ --														
360	1:10	AIR									474	475:50	4.5	
		AIR/O_2									118	134:50		

Appendix

(DESCENT RATE 75 FPM—ASCENT RATE 30 FPM)

Bottom Time (min)	Time to First Stop (M:S)	Gas Mix	DECOMPRESSION STOPS (FSW) Stop times (min) include travel time, except first air and first O₂ stop									Total Ascent Time (M:S)	Chamber O₂ Periods	Repet Group
			100	90	80	70	60	50	40	30	20			
60 FSW														
60	2:00	AIR									0	2:00	0	K
		AIR/O₂									0	2:00		
65	1:20	AIR									2	4:00	0.5	L
		AIR/O₂									1	3:00		
70	1:20	AIR									7	9:00	0.5	L
		AIR/O₂									4	6:00		
80	1:20	AIR									14	16:00	0.5	N
		AIR/O₂									7	9:00		
In-Water Air/O₂ Decompression or SurDO₂ Recommended --															
90	1:20	AIR									23	25:00	0.5	O
		AIR/O₂									10	12:00		
100	1:20	AIR									42	44:00	1	Z
		AIR/O₂									15	17:00		
110	1:20	AIR									57	59:00	1	Z
		AIR/O₂									21	23:00		
120	1:20	AIR									75	77:00	1	Z
		AIR/O₂									26	28:00		
Exceptional Exposure: In-Water Air Decompression ------------- In-Water Air/O₂ Decompression or SurDO₂ Required ----------															
130	1:20	AIR									102	104:00	1.5	Z
		AIR/O₂									31	33:00		
140	1:20	AIR									124	126:00	1.5	Z
		AIR/O₂									35	37:00		
150	1:20	AIR									143	145:00	2	Z
		AIR/O₂									41	48:00		
160	1:20	AIR									158	160:00	2	Z
		AIR/O₂									48	55:00		
170	1:20	AIR									178	180:00	2	
		AIR/O₂									53	60:00		
180	1:20	AIR									201	203:00	2.5	
		AIR/O₂									59	66:00		
190	1:20	AIR									222	224:00	2.5	
		AIR/O₂									64	71:00		
200	1:20	AIR									240	242:00	2.5	
		AIR/O₂									68	80:00		
210	1:20	AIR									256	258:00	3	
		AIR/O₂									73	85:00		
220	1:20	AIR									278	280:00	3	
		AIR/O₂									77	89:00		
Exceptional Exposure: In-Water Air/O₂ Decompression ------------- SurDO₂ Required--------------------------------------															
230	1:20	AIR									300	302:00	3.5	
		AIR/O₂									82	94:00		
240	1:20	AIR									321	323:00	3.5	
		AIR/O₂									88	100:00		
270	1:20	AIR									398	400:00	4	
		AIR/O₂									102	119:00		
Exceptional Exposure: SurDO₂ --															
300	1:20	AIR									456	458:00	4.5	
		AIR/O₂									115	132:00		

Appendix

(DESCENT RATE 75 FPM—ASCENT RATE 30 FPM)

Bottom Time (min)	Time to First Stop (M:S)	Gas Mix	DECOMPRESSION STOPS (FSW) Stop times (min) include travel time, except first air and first O₂ stop									Total Ascent Time (M:S)	Chamber O₂ Periods	Repet Group
			100	90	80	70	60	50	40	30	20			
70 FSW														
48	2:20	AIR									0	2:20	0	K
		AIR/O₂									0	2:20		
50	1:40	AIR									2	4:20	0.5	K
		AIR/O₂									1	3:20		
55	1:40	AIR									9	11:20	0.5	L
		AIR/O₂									5	7:20		
60	1:40	AIR									14	16:20	0.5	M
		AIR/O₂									8	10:20		
In-Water Air/O₂ Decompression or SurDO₂ Recommended														
70	1:40	AIR									24	26:20	0.5	N
		AIR/O₂									13	15:20		
80	1:40	AIR									44	46:20	1	O
		AIR/O₂									17	19:20		
90	1:40	AIR									64	66:20	1	Z
		AIR/O₂									24	26:20		
100	1:40	AIR									88	90:20	1.5	Z
		AIR/O₂									31	33:20		
Exceptional Exposure: In-Water Air Decompression ———— In-Water Air/O₂ Decompression or SurDO₂ Required														
110	1:40	AIR									120	122:20	1.5	Z
		AIR/O₂									38	45:20		
120	1:40	AIR									145	147:20	2	Z
		AIR/O₂									44	51:20		
130	1:40	AIR									167	169:20	2	Z
		AIR/O₂									51	58:20		
140	1:40	AIR									189	191:20	2.5	
		AIR/O₂									59	66:20		
150	1:40	AIR									219	221:20	2.5	
		AIR/O₂									66	78:20		
160	1:20	AIR								1	244	247:00	3	
		AIR/O₂								1	72	85:00		
Exceptional Exposure: In-Water Air/O₂ Decompression ———— SurDO₂ Required														
170	1:20	AIR								2	265	269:00	3	
		AIR/O₂								1	78	91:00		
180	1:20	AIR								4	289	295:00	3.5	
		AIR/O₂								2	83	97:00		
190	1:20	AIR								5	316	323:00	3.5	
		AIR/O₂								3	88	103:00		
200	1:20	AIR								9	345	356:00	4	
		AIR/O₂								5	93	115:00		
210	1:20	AIR								13	378	393:00	4	
		AIR/O₂								7	98	122:00		
Exceptional Exposure: SurDO₂														
240	1:20	AIR								25	454	481:00	5	
		AIR/O₂								13	110	140:00		

Appendix

(DESCENT RATE 75 FPM—ASCENT RATE 30 FPM)

Bottom Time (min)	Time to First Stop (M:S)	Gas Mix	DECOMPRESSION STOPS (FSW) Stop times (min) include travel time, except first air and first O₂ stop									Total Ascent Time (M:S)	Chamber O₂ Periods	Repet Group
			100	90	80	70	60	50	40	30	20			
80 FSW														
39	2:40	AIR									0	2:40	0	J
		AIR/O₂									0	2:40		
40	2:00	AIR									1	3:40	0.5	J
		AIR/O₂									1	3:40		
45	2:00	AIR									10	12:40	0.5	K
		AIR/O₂									5	7:40		
In-Water Air/O₂ Decompression or SurDO₂ Recommended															
50	2:00	AIR									17	19:40	0.5	M
		AIR/O₂									9	11:40		
55	2:00	AIR									24	26:40	0.5	M
		AIR/O₂									13	15:40		
60	2:00	AIR									30	32:40	1	N
		AIR/O₂									16	18:40		
70	2:00	AIR									54	56:40	1	O
		AIR/O₂									22	24:40		
80	2:00	AIR									77	79:40	1.5	Z
		AIR/O₂									30	32:40		
Exceptional Exposure: In-Water Air Decompression ———— In-Water Air/O₂ Decompression or SurDO₂ Required															
90	2:00	AIR									114	116:40	1.5	Z
		AIR/O₂									39	46:40		
100	1:40	AIR								1	147	150:20	2	Z
		AIR/O₂								1	46	54:20		
110	1:40	AIR								6	171	179:20	2	Z
		AIR/O₂								3	51	61:20		
120	1:40	AIR								10	200	212:20	2.5	
		AIR/O₂								5	59	71:20		
130	1:40	AIR								14	232	248:20	3	
		AIR/O₂								7	67	86:20		
Exceptional Exposure: In-Water Air/O₂ Decompression ———— SurDO₂ Required															
140	1:40	AIR								17	258	277:20	3.5	
		AIR/O₂								9	73	94:20		
150	1:40	AIR								19	285	306:20	3.5	
		AIR/O₂								10	80	102:20		
160	1:40	AIR								21	318	341:20	4	
		AIR/O₂								11	86	114:20		
170	1:40	AIR								27	354	383:20	4	
		AIR/O₂								14	90	121:20		
Exceptional Exposure: SurDO₂															
180	1:40	AIR								33	391	426:20	4.5	
		AIR/O₂								17	96	130:20		
210	1:40	AIR								50	474	526:20	5	
		AIR/O₂								26	110	158:20		

Appendix

(DESCENT RATE 75 FPM—ASCENT RATE 30 FPM)

Bottom Time (min)	Time to First Stop (M:S)	Gas Mix	\multicolumn{8}{c	}{DECOMPRESSION STOPS (FSW) Stop times (min) include travel time, except first air and first O₂ stop}	Total Ascent Time (M:S)	Chamber O₂ Periods	Repet Group
			100	90	80	70	60	50	40	30	20			

90 FSW

Bottom Time (min)	Time to First Stop (M:S)	Gas Mix	100	90	80	70	60	50	40	30	20	Total Ascent Time (M:S)	Chamber O₂ Periods	Repet Group
30	3:00	AIR									0	3:00	0	I
		AIR/O₂									0	3:00		
35	2:20	AIR									4	7:00	0.5	J
		AIR/O₂									2	5:00		
40	2:20	AIR									14	17:00	0.5	L
		AIR/O₂									7	10:00		
\multicolumn{14}{	l	}{In-Water Air/O₂ Decompression or SurDO₂ Recommended}
45	2:20	AIR									23	26:00	0.5	M
		AIR/O₂									12	15:00		
50	2:20	AIR									31	34:00	1	N
		AIR/O₂									17	20:00		
55	2:20	AIR									39	42:00	1	O
		AIR/O₂									21	24:00		
60	2:20	AIR									56	59:00	1	O
		AIR/O₂									24	27:00		
70	2:20	AIR									83	86:00	1.5	Z
		AIR/O₂									32	35:00		
\multicolumn{14}{	l	}{Exceptional Exposure: In-Water Air Decompression ------------ In-Water Air/O₂ Decompression or SurDO₂ Required}
80	2:00	AIR								5	125	132:40	2	Z
		AIR/O₂								3	40	50:40		
90	2:00	AIR								13	158	173:40	2	Z
		AIR/O₂								7	46	60:40		
100	2:00	AIR								19	185	206:40	2.5	
		AIR/O₂								10	53	70:40		
110	2:00	AIR								25	224	251:40	3	
		AIR/O₂								13	61	86:40		
\multicolumn{14}{	l	}{Exceptional Exposure: In-Water Air/O₂ Decompression ------------ SurDO₂ Required}
120	1:40	AIR							1	29	256	288:20	3.5	
		AIR/O₂							1	15	70	98:40		
130	1:40	AIR							5	28	291	326:20	3.5	
		AIR/O₂							5	15	78	110:40		
140	1:40	AIR							8	28	330	368:20	4	
		AIR/O₂							8	15	86	126:40		
\multicolumn{14}{	l	}{Exceptional Exposure: SurDO₂}
150	1:40	AIR							11	34	378	425:20	4.5	
		AIR/O₂							11	17	94	139:40		
160	1:40	AIR							13	40	418	473:20	4.5	
		AIR/O₂							13	21	100	151:40		
170	1:40	AIR							15	45	451	513:20	5	
		AIR/O₂							15	23	106	166:40		
180	1:40	AIR							16	51	479	548:20	5.5	
		AIR/O₂							16	26	112	176:40		
240	1:40	AIR							42	68	592	704:20	7.5	
		AIR/O₂							42	34	159	267:00		

Appendix

(DESCENT RATE 75 FPM—ASCENT RATE 30 FPM)

100 FSW

Bottom Time (min)	Time to First Stop (M:S)	Gas Mix	DECOMPRESSION STOPS (FSW) Stop times (min) include travel time, except first air and first O_2 stop									Total Ascent Time (M:S)	Chamber O_2 Periods	Repet Group
			100	90	80	70	60	50	40	30	20			
25	3:20	AIR										0	3:20	0	H
		AIR/O_2										0	3:20		
30	2:40	AIR										3	6:20	0.5	J
		AIR/O_2										2	5:20		
35	2:40	AIR										15	18:20	0.5	L
		AIR/O_2										8	11:20		
In-Water Air/O_2 Decompression or SurDO$_2$ Recommended															
40	2:40	AIR										26	29:20	1	M
		AIR/O_2										14	17:20		
45	2:40	AIR										36	39:20	1	N
		AIR/O_2										19	22:20		
50	2:40	AIR										47	50:20	1	O
		AIR/O_2										24	27:20		
55	2:40	AIR										65	68:20	1.5	Z
		AIR/O_2										28	31:20		
60	2:40	AIR										81	84:20	1.5	Z
		AIR/O_2										33	35:20		
Exceptional Exposure: In-Water Air Decompression -------- In-Water Air/O_2 Decompression or SurDO$_2$ Required															
70	2:20	AIR									11	124	138:00	2	Z
		AIR/O_2									6	39	53:00		
80	2:20	AIR									21	160	184:00	2.5	Z
		AIR/O_2									11	45	64:00		
90	2:00	AIR								2	28	196	228:40	2.5	
		AIR/O_2								2	15	52	82:00		
Exceptional Exposure: In-Water Air/O_2 Decompression ------- SurDO$_2$ Required															
100	2:00	AIR								9	28	241	280:40	3	
		AIR/O_2								9	14	66	102:00		
110	2:00	AIR								14	28	278	322:40	3.5	
		AIR/O_2								14	15	75	117:00		
120	2:00	AIR								19	28	324	373:40	4	
		AIR/O_2								19	15	84	136:00		
Exceptional Exposure: SurDO$_2$															
150	1:40	AIR							3	26	46	461	538:20	5	
		AIR/O_2							3	26	24	108	183:40		

Appendix

(DESCENT RATE 75 FPM—ASCENT RATE 30 FPM)

110 FSW

Bottom Time (min)	Time to First Stop (M:S)	Gas Mix	\multicolumn{8}{c}{DECOMPRESSION STOPS (FSW) Stop times (min) include travel time, except first air and first O_2 stop}	Total Ascent Time (M:S)	Chamber O_2 Periods	Repet Group
			100	90	80	70	60	50	40	30	20			
20	3:40	AIR									0	3:40	0	H
		AIR/O_2									0	3:40		
25	3:00	AIR									3	6:40	0.5	I
		AIR/O_2									2	5:40		
30	3:00	AIR									14	17:40	0.5	K
		AIR/O_2									7	10:40		
\multicolumn{14}{l}{In-Water Air/O_2 Decompression or SurDO$_2$ Recommended}
35	3:00	AIR									27	30:40	1	M
		AIR/O_2									14	17:40		
40	3:00	AIR									39	42:40	1	N
		AIR/O_2									20	23:40		
45	3:00	AIR									50	53:40	1	O
		AIR/O_2									26	29:40		
50	3:00	AIR									71	74:40	1.5	Z
		AIR/O_2									31	34:40		
\multicolumn{14}{l}{Exceptional Exposure: In-Water Air Decompression ------------ In-Water Air/O_2 Decompression or SurDO$_2$ Required}
55	2:40	AIR								5	85	93:20	1.5	Z
		AIR/O_2								3	33	44:20		
60	2:40	AIR								13	111	127:20	2	Z
		AIR/O_2								7	36	51:20		
70	2:40	AIR								26	155	184:20	2.5	Z
		AIR/O_2								13	43	64:20		
80	2:20	AIR								9	28	200	240:00	2.5	
		AIR/O_2								9	15	53	90:20		
\multicolumn{14}{l}{Exceptional Exposure: In-Water Air/O_2 Decompression ------------ SurDO$_2$ Required}
90	2:20	AIR							17	29	248	297:00	3.5	
		AIR/O_2							17	15	67	112:20		
100	2:20	AIR							25	28	295	351:00	3.5	
		AIR/O_2							25	15	78	131:20		
110	2:00	AIR						5	26	28	353	414:40	4	
		AIR/O_2						5	26	15	90	154:00		
\multicolumn{14}{l}{Exceptional Exposure: SurDO$_2$}
120	2:00	AIR						10	26	35	413	486:40	4.5	
		AIR/O_2						10	26	18	101	173:00		
180	1:40	AIR					3	23	47	68	593	736:20	7.5	
		AIR/O_2					3	23	47	34	159	298:00		

Appendix

(DESCENT RATE 75 FPM—ASCENT RATE 30 FPM)

120 FSW

Bottom Time (min)	Time to First Stop (M:S)	Gas Mix	Decompression Stops (FSW) 100	90	80	70	60	50	40	30	20	Total Ascent Time (M:S)	Chamber O₂ Periods	Repet Group
15	4:00	AIR										0 / 4:00	0	F
		AIR/O₂										0 / 4:00		
20	3:20	AIR										2 / 6:00	0.5	H
		AIR/O₂										1 / 5:00		
25	3:20	AIR										8 / 12:00	0.5	J
		AIR/O₂										4 / 8:00		
In-Water Air/O₂ Decompression or SurDO₂ Recommended															
30	3:20	AIR										24 / 28:00	0.5	L
		AIR/O₂										13 / 17:00		
35	3:20	AIR										38 / 42:00	1	N
		AIR/O₂										20 / 24:00		
40	3:20	AIR										51 / 55:00	1	O
		AIR/O₂										27 / 31:00		
45	3:20	AIR										72 / 76:00	1.5	Z
		AIR/O₂										33 / 37:00		
Exceptional Exposure: In-Water Air Decompression ------- In-Water Air/O₂ Decompression or SurDO₂ Required															
50	3:00	AIR									9	86 / 98:40	1.5	Z
		AIR/O₂									5	33 / 46:40		
55	3:00	AIR									19	116 / 138:40	2	Z
		AIR/O₂									10	35 / 53:40		
60	3:00	AIR									27	142 / 172:40	2	Z
		AIR/O₂									14	39 / 61:40		
70	2:40	AIR								12	29	189 / 233:20	2.5	
		AIR/O₂								12	15	50 / 85:40		
Exceptional Exposure: In-Water Air/O₂ Decompression ------- SurDO₂ Required															
80	2:40	AIR								24	28	246 / 301:20	3	
		AIR/O₂								24	14	67 / 118:40		
90	2:20	AIR							7	26	28	303 / 367:00	3.5	
		AIR/O₂							7	26	15	79 / 140:20		
100	2:20	AIR							14	26	28	372 / 443:00	4	
		AIR/O₂							14	26	15	94 / 167:20		
Exceptional Exposure: SurDO₂															
110	2:20	AIR							21	25	38	433 / 520:00	5	
		AIR/O₂							21	25	20	104 / 188:20		
120	2:00	AIR						3	23	25	47	480 / 580:40	5.5	
		AIR/O₂						3	23	25	24	113 / 211:00		

Appendix

(DESCENT RATE 75 FPM—ASCENT RATE 30 FPM)

130 FSW

Bottom Time (min)	Time to First Stop (M:S)	Gas Mix	\multicolumn{8}{c}{DECOMPRESSION STOPS (FSW) Stop times (min) include travel time, except first air and first O₂ stop}	Total Ascent Time (M:S)	Chamber O₂ Periods	Repet Group
			100	90	80	70	60	50	40	30	20			
10	4:20	AIR									0	4:20	0	E
		AIR/O$_2$									0	4:20		
15	3:40	AIR									1	5:20	0.5	G
		AIR/O$_2$									1	5:20		
20	3:40	AIR									4	8:20	0.5	I
		AIR/O$_2$									2	6:20		
\multicolumn{14}{l}{In-Water Air/O$_2$ Decompression or SurDO$_2$ Recommended}
25	3:40	AIR									17	21:20	0.5	K
		AIR/O$_2$									9	13:20		
30	3:40	AIR									34	38:20	1	M
		AIR/O$_2$									18	22:20		
35	3:40	AIR									49	53:20	1	N
		AIR/O$_2$									26	30:20		
40	3:20	AIR								3	67	74:00	1.5	Z
		AIR/O$_2$								2	31	37:00		
\multicolumn{14}{l}{Exceptional Exposure: In-Water Air Decompression ---------- In-Water Air/O$_2$ Decompression or SurDO$_2$ Required ----------}
45	3:20	AIR								12	84	100:00	1.5	Z
		AIR/O$_2$								6	33	48:00		
50	3:20	AIR								22	116	142:00	2	Z
		AIR/O$_2$								11	35	55:00		
55	3:00	AIR							4	28	145	180:40	2	Z
		AIR/O$_2$							4	15	39	67:00		
60	3:00	AIR							12	28	170	213:40	2.5	Z
		AIR/O$_2$							12	15	45	81:00		
\multicolumn{14}{l}{Exceptional Exposure: In-Water Air/O$_2$ Decompression ---------- SurDO$_2$ Required----------}
70	2:40	AIR						1	26	28	235	293:20	3	
		AIR/O$_2$						1	26	14	63	117:40		
80	2:40	AIR						12	26	28	297	366:20	3.5	
		AIR/O$_2$						12	26	15	78	144:40		
90	2:40	AIR						21	26	28	374	452:20	4	
		AIR/O$_2$						21	26	15	94	174:40		
\multicolumn{14}{l}{Exceptional Exposure: SurDO$_2$ ----------}
100	2:20	AIR					6	23	26	38	444	540:00	5	
		AIR/O$_2$					6	23	26	20	106	204:20		
120	2:20	AIR					17	23	28	57	533	661:00	6	
		AIR/O$_2$					17	23	28	29	130	255:20		
180	2:00	AIR				13	21	45	57	94	658	890:40	9	
		AIR/O$_2$				13	21	45	57	46	198	417:20		

Appendix

(DESCENT RATE 75 FPM—ASCENT RATE 30 FPM)

140 FSW

Bottom Time (min)	Time to First Stop (M:S)	Gas Mix	\multicolumn{8}{c}{DECOMPRESSION STOPS (FSW) Stop times (min) include travel time, except first air and first O_2 stop}	Total Ascent Time (M:S)	Chamber O_2 Periods	Repet Group

Bottom Time (min)	Time to First Stop (M:S)	Gas Mix	100	90	80	70	60	50	40	30	20	Total Ascent Time (M:S)	Chamber O_2 Periods	Repet Group
10	4:40	AIR									0	4:40	0	E
		AIR/O_2									0	4:40		
15	4:00	AIR									2	6:40	0.5	H
		AIR/O_2									1	5:40		
20	4:00	AIR									7	11:40	0.5	J
		AIR/O_2									4	8:40		
\multicolumn{15}{l}{In-Water Air/O_2 Decompression or SurDO_2 Recommended}
25	4:00	AIR									26	30:40	1	L
		AIR/O_2									14	18:40		
30	4:00	AIR									44	48:40	1	N
		AIR/O_2									23	27:40		
35	3:40	AIR								4	59	67:20	1.5	O
		AIR/O_2								2	30	36:20		
\multicolumn{15}{l}{Exceptional Exposure: In-Water Air Decompression ------- In-Water Air/O_2 Decompression or SurDO_2 Required}
40	3:40	AIR								11	80	95:20	1.5	Z
		AIR/O_2								6	33	48:20		
45	3:20	AIR							3	21	113	141:00	2	Z
		AIR/O_2							3	11	34	57:20		
50	3:20	AIR							7	28	145	184:00	2	Z
		AIR/O_2							7	14	40	70:20		
55	3:20	AIR							16	28	171	219:00	2.5	Z
		AIR/O_2							16	15	45	85:20		
\multicolumn{15}{l}{Exceptional Exposure: In-Water Air/O_2 Decompression ------- SurDO_2 Required}
60	3:00	AIR						2	23	28	209	265:40	3	
		AIR/O_2						2	23	15	55	109:00		
70	3:00	AIR					14	25	28	276	346:40	3.5		
		AIR/O_2					14	25	15	74	142:00			
80	2:40	AIR				2	24	25	29	362	446:20	4		
		AIR/O_2				2	24	25	15	91	175:40			
\multicolumn{15}{l}{Exceptional Exposure: SurDO_2}
90	2:40	AIR				12	23	26	38	443	545:20	5		
		AIR/O_2				12	23	26	19	107	210:40			

Appendix

(DESCENT RATE 75 FPM—ASCENT RATE 30 FPM)

Bottom Time (min)	Time to First Stop (M:S)	Gas Mix	DECOMPRESSION STOPS (FSW) Stop times (min) include travel time, except first air and first O_2 stop									Total Ascent Time (M:S)	Chamber O_2 Periods	Repet Group
			100	90	80	70	60	50	40	30	20			
150 FSW														
5	5:00	AIR									0	5:00	0	C
		AIR/O_2									0	5:00		
10	4:20	AIR									1	6:00	0.5	F
		AIR/O_2									1	6:00		
15	4:20	AIR									3	8:00	0.5	H
		AIR/O_2									2	7:00		
20	4:20	AIR									14	19:00	0.5	K
		AIR/O_2									8	13:00		
In-Water Air/O_2 Decompression or SurDO_2 Recommended														
25	4:20	AIR									35	40:00	1	M
		AIR/O_2									19	24:00		
30	4:00	AIR								3	51	58:40	1.5	O
		AIR/O_2								2	26	32:40		
35	4:00	AIR								11	72	87:40	1.5	Z
		AIR/O_2								6	31	46:40		
Exceptional Exposure: In-Water Air Decompression ———— In-Water Air/O_2 Decompression or SurDO_2 Required														
40	3:40	AIR							4	18	102	128:20	2	Z
		AIR/O_2							4	9	34	56:40		
45	3:40	AIR							10	25	140	179:20	2	Z
		AIR/O_2							10	13	39	71:40		
50	3:20	AIR						3	15	28	170	220:00	2.5	Z
		AIR/O_2						3	15	15	45	87:20		
Exceptional Exposure: In-Water Air/O_2 Decompression ———— SurDO_2 Required														
55	3:20	AIR						6	22	28	211	271:00	3	
		AIR/O_2						6	22	15	56	113:20		
60	3:20	AIR						11	26	28	248	317:00	3	
		AIR/O_2						11	26	15	66	132:20		
70	3:00	AIR					3	24	25	28	330	413:40	4	
		AIR/O_2					3	24	25	15	84	170:00		
Exceptional Exposure: SurDO_2														
80	3:00	AIR					15	23	26	35	430	532:40	4.5	
		AIR/O_2					15	23	26	18	104	205:00		
90	2:40	AIR				3	22	23	26	47	496	620:20	5.5	
		AIR/O_2				3	22	23	26	24	118	239:40		
120	2:20	AIR			3	20	22	23	50	75	608	804:00	8	
		AIR/O_2			3	20	22	23	50	37	168	355:40		
180	2:00	AIR	2	19	20	42	48	79	121	694	1027:40	10.5		
		AIR/O_2	2	19	20	42	48	79	58	222	537:20			

Appendix

(DESCENT RATE 75 FPM—ASCENT RATE 30 FPM)

Bottom Time (min)	Time to First Stop (M:S)	Gas Mix	\multicolumn{9}{c}{DECOMPRESSION STOPS (FSW) — Stop times (min) include travel time, except first air and first O₂ stop}	Total Ascent Time (M:S)	Chamber O₂ Periods	Repet Group
			100	90	80	70	60	50	40	30	20			
160 FSW														
5	5:20	AIR										0	5:20	0	C
		AIR/O₂										0	5:20		
10	4:40	AIR										1	6:20	0.5	F
		AIR/O₂										1	6:20		
15	4:40	AIR										5	10:20	0.5	I
		AIR/O₂										3	8:00		
In-Water Air/O₂ Decompression or SurDO₂ Recommended															
20	4:40	AIR										22	27:20	0.5	L
		AIR/O₂										12	17:20		
25	4:20	AIR									3	41	49:00	1	N
		AIR/O₂									2	21	28:00		
30	4:00	AIR								1	8	60	73:40	1.5	O
		AIR/O₂								1	5	28	39:00		
Exceptional Exposure: In-Water Air Decompression ——— In-Water Air/O₂ Decompression or SurDO₂ Required															
35	4:00	AIR								4	14	84	106:40	1.5	Z
		AIR/O₂								4	8	32	54:00		
40	4:00	AIR								12	20	130	166:40	2	Z
		AIR/O₂								12	11	37	70:00		
45	3:40	AIR							5	13	28	164	214:20	2.5	Z
		AIR/O₂							5	13	14	44	85:40		
Exceptional Exposure: In-Water Air/O₂ Decompression ——— SurDO₂ Required															
50	3:40	AIR						10	19	28	207		268:20	3	
		AIR/O₂						10	19	15	54		112:40		
55	3:20	AIR					2	12	26	28	248		320:00	3	
		AIR/O₂					2	12	26	14	67		135:20		
60	3:20	AIR					5	18	25	29	290		371:00	3.5	
		AIR/O₂					5	18	25	15	77		154:20		
Exceptional Exposure: SurDO₂															
70	3:20	AIR					15	23	26	29	399		496:00	4.5	
		AIR/O₂					15	23	26	15	99		197:20		
80	3:00	AIR				6	21	24	25	44	482		605:40	5.5	
		AIR/O₂				6	21	24	25	23	114		237:00		

Appendix

(DESCENT RATE 75 FPM—ASCENT RATE 30 FPM)

170 FSW

Bottom Time (min)	Time to First Stop (M:S)	Gas Mix	\multicolumn{8}{c}{DECOMPRESSION STOPS (FSW) — Stop times (min) include travel time, except first air and first O₂ stop}								Total Ascent Time (M:S)	Chamber O₂ Periods	Repet Group
			100	90	80	70	60	50	40	30	20			
5	5:40	AIR									0	5:40	0	D
		AIR/O₂									0	5:40		
10	5:00	AIR									2	7:40	0.5	G
		AIR/O₂									1	6:40		
15	5:00	AIR									7	12:40	0.5	J
		AIR/O₂									4	9:40		
In-Water Air/O₂ Decompression or SurDO₂ Recommended														
20	4:40	AIR								1	29	35:20	1	L
		AIR/O₂								1	15	21:20		
25	4:20	AIR							1	6	46	58:00	1	N
		AIR/O₂							1	4	23	33:20		
Exceptional Exposure: In-Water Air Decompression ---- In-Water Air/O₂ Decompression or SurDO₂ Required														
30	4:20	AIR							5	11	72	93:00	1.5	Z
		AIR/O₂							5	6	29	45:20		
35	4:00	AIR						2	9	17	113	145:40	2	Z
		AIR/O₂						2	9	9	35	65:00		
40	4:00	AIR						6	13	23	155	201:40	2.5	Z
		AIR/O₂						6	13	12	43	84:00		
Exceptional Exposure: In-Water Air/O₂ Decompression ---- SurDO₂ Required														
45	4:00	AIR						12	16	28	194	254:40	2.5	
		AIR/O₂						12	16	15	51	109:00		
50	3:40	AIR					5	12	23	28	243	315:20	3	
		AIR/O₂					5	12	23	15	65	134:40		
55	3:40	AIR					9	16	25	28	287	369:20	3.5	
		AIR/O₂					9	16	25	15	76	155:40		
60	3:20	AIR				2	11	21	26	28	344	436:00	4	
		AIR/O₂				2	11	21	26	15	87	181:20		
Exceptional Exposure: SurDO₂														
70	3:20	AIR				7	19	24	25	39	454	572:00	5	
		AIR/O₂				7	19	24	25	20	109	228:20		
80	3:20	AIR				17	22	23	26	53	525	670:00	6	
		AIR/O₂				17	22	23	26	27	128	267:20		
90	3:00	AIR			7	20	22	23	37	66	574	752:40	7	
		AIR/O₂			7	20	22	23	37	33	148	318:20		
120	2:40	AIR		9	19	20	22	42	60	94	659	928:20	9	
		AIR/O₂		9	19	20	22	42	60	46	198	454:00		
180	2:20	AIR	10	18	19	40	43	70	97	156	703	1159:00	11.5	
		AIR/O₂	10	18	19	40	43	70	97	75	228	648:00		

Appendix

(DESCENT RATE 75 FPM—ASCENT RATE 30 FPM)

180 FSW

Bottom Time (min)	Time to First Stop (M:S)	Gas Mix	100	90	80	70	60	50	40	30	20	Total Ascent Time (M:S)	Chamber O_2 Periods	Repet Group
5	6:00	AIR									0	6:00	0	D
		AIR/O_2									0	6:00		
10	5:20	AIR									3	9:00	0.5	G
		AIR/O_2									2	8:00		
15	5:20	AIR									11	17:00	0.5	J
		AIR/O_2									6	12:00		
In-Water Air/O_2 Decompression or SurDO_2 Recommended															
20	5:00	AIR								4	34	43:40	1	M
		AIR/O_2								2	18	25:40		
25	4:40	AIR							4	7	54	70:20	1.5	O
		AIR/O_2							4	4	26	39:40		
Exceptional Exposure: In-Water Air Decompression ———— In-Water Air/O_2 Decompression or SurDO_2 Required															
30	4:20	AIR						2	7	14	83	111:00	1.5	Z
		AIR/O_2						2	7	7	31	57:20		
35	4:20	AIR						5	13	19	138	180:00	2	Z
		AIR/O_2						5	13	10	40	78:20		
Exceptional Exposure: In-Water Air/O_2 Decompression ———— SurDO_2 Required															
40	4:00	AIR					2	11	12	28	175	232:40	2.5	Z
		AIR/O_2					2	11	12	14	47	96:00		
45	4:00	AIR					7	11	20	28	231	301:40	3	
		AIR/O_2					7	11	20	15	61	129:00		
50	3:40	AIR				1	11	13	25	28	276	358:20	3.5	
		AIR/O_2				1	11	13	25	15	74	153:40		
55	3:40	AIR				5	11	19	26	28	336	429:20	4	
		AIR/O_2				5	11	19	26	14	87	181:40		
Exceptional Exposure: SurDO_2															
60	3:40	AIR				8	13	24	25	31	405	510:20	4.5	
		AIR/O_2				8	13	24	25	16	100	205:40		
70	3:20	AIR			3	13	21	24	25	48	498	636:00	5.5	
		AIR/O_2			3	13	21	24	25	25	118	253:20		

Appendix

(DESCENT RATE 75 FPM—ASCENT RATE 30 FPM)

Bottom Time (min)	Time to First Stop (M:S)	Gas Mix	DECOMPRESSION STOPS (FSW) Stop times (min) include travel time, except first air and first O₂ stop									Total Ascent Time (M:S)	Chamber O₂ Periods	Repet Group
			100	90	80	70	60	50	40	30	20			

190 FSW

Bottom Time	First Stop	Gas Mix	100	90	80	70	60	50	40	30	20	Total Ascent	O₂ Periods	Repet
5	6:20	AIR									0	6:20	0	D
		AIR/O₂									0	6:20		
10	5:40	AIR									4	10:20	0.5	H
		AIR/O₂									2	8:20		
In-Water Air/O₂ Decompression or SurDO₂ Recommended														
15	5:40	AIR									17	23:20	0.5	K
		AIR/O₂									9	15:20		
20	5:00	AIR							1	7	37	50:40	1	N
		AIR/O₂							1	4	19	30:00		
25	4:40	AIR						2	6	9	67	89:20	1.5	Z
		AIR/O₂						2	6	5	28	46:40		
Exceptional Exposure: In-Water Air Decompression ----- In-Water Air/O₂ Decompression or SurDO₂ Required														
30	4:40	AIR					6	8	14	111		144:20	2	Z
		AIR/O₂					6	8	8	35		67:40		
35	4:20	AIR				3	8	13	22	160		211:00	2.5	Z
		AIR/O₂				3	8	13	12	44		90:20		
Exceptional Exposure: In-Water Air/O₂ Decompression ----- SurDO₂ Required														
40	4:20	AIR				7	12	14	29	210		277:00	3	
		AIR/O₂				7	12	14	15	56		119:20		
45	4:00	AIR			2	11	12	23	28	262		342:40	3.5	
		AIR/O₂			2	11	12	23	15	70		148:00		
50	4:00	AIR			7	11	16	26	28	321		413:40	4	
		AIR/O₂			7	11	16	26	15	83		178:00		
Exceptional Exposure: SurDO2														
55	3:40	AIR			2	10	10	24	25	30	396	501:20	4.5	
		AIR/O₂			2	10	10	24	25	16	98	204:40		
60	3:40	AIR			5	10	16	24	25	40	454	578:20	5	
		AIR/O₂			5	10	16	24	25	21	108	233:40		
90	3:20	AIR		11	19	20	21	28	51	83	626	863:00	8.5	
		AIR/O₂		11	19	20	21	28	51	42	177	408:40		
120	3:00	AIR	15	17	19	20	37	46	79	113	691	1040:40	10.5	
		AIR/O₂	15	17	19	20	37	46	79	55	219	550:20		

Appendix

(DESCENT RATE 75 FPM—ASCENT RATE 30 FPM)

200 FSW

Exceptional Exposure

Bottom Time (min)	Time to First Stop (M:S)	Gas Mix	100	90	80	70	60	50	40	30	20	Total Ascent Time (M:S)	Chamber O₂ Periods	Repet Group
5	6:00	AIR									1	7:40	0.5	
		AIR/O₂									1	7:40		
10	6:00	AIR									2	8:40	0.5	
		AIR/O₂									1	7:40		
15	5:40	AIR								2	22	30:20	0.5	
		AIR/O₂								1	11	18:20		
20	5:20	AIR							5	6	43	60:00	1	
		AIR/O₂							5	4	21	36:20		
25	5:00	AIR						5	6	11	78	105:40	1.5	
		AIR/O₂						5	6	6	29	52:00		
30	4:40	AIR					4	5	11	18	136	179:20	2	
		AIR/O₂					4	5	11	9	40	79:40		
35	4:20	AIR				1	6	10	13	26	179	240:00	2.5	
		AIR/O₂				1	6	10	13	13	49	102:20		
40	4:20	AIR				3	10	12	18	28	243	319:00	3	
		AIR/O₂				3	10	12	18	15	65	138:20		
45	4:20	AIR				8	11	12	26	28	300	390:00	3.5	
		AIR/O₂				8	11	12	26	15	79	166:20		
50	4:00	AIR			3	10	11	20	26	28	377	479:40	4.5	
		AIR/O₂			3	10	11	20	26	15	95	200:00		

210 FSW

Exceptional Exposure

Bottom Time (min)	Time to First Stop (M:S)	Gas Mix	100	90	80	70	60	50	40	30	20	Total Ascent Time (M:S)	Chamber O₂ Periods	Repet Group
5	6:20	AIR									1	8:00	0.5	
		AIR/O₂									1	8:00		
10	6:20	AIR									5	12:00	0.5	
		AIR/O₂									3	10:00		
15	6:00	AIR								5	26	37:40	1	
		AIR/O₂								3	13	22:40		
20	5:20	AIR						2	6	7	50	71:00	1.5	
		AIR/O₂						2	6	4	24	42:20		
25	5:00	AIR					2	6	7	13	94	127:40	1.5	
		AIR/O₂					2	6	7	7	32	65:00		
30	4:40	AIR				2	5	6	13	21	156	208:20	2	
		AIR/O₂				2	5	6	13	11	43	90:40		
35	4:40	AIR				5	6	12	14	28	214	284:20	3	
		AIR/O₂				5	6	12	14	14	58	124:40		
40	4:20	AIR			2	6	11	12	22	28	271	357:00	3.5	
		AIR/O₂			2	6	11	12	22	15	74	157:20		
45	4:20	AIR			4	10	11	16	25	29	347	447:00	4	
		AIR/O₂			4	10	11	16	25	15	89	190:20		
50	4:20	AIR			9	10	11	23	26	35	426	545:00	4.5	
		AIR/O₂			9	10	11	23	26	18	104	221:20		

Appendix

(DESCENT RATE 75 FPM—ASCENT RATE 30 FPM)

Bottom Time (min)	Time to First Stop (M:S)	Gas Mix	DECOMPRESSION STOPS (FSW) Stop times (min) include travel time, except first air and first O₂ stop								Total Ascent Time (M:S)	Chamber O₂ Periods	Repet Group
			100	90	80	70	60	50	40	30	20			

220 FSW
Exceptional Exposure

Bottom Time	Time to First Stop	Gas Mix	100	90	80	70	60	50	40	30	20	Total Ascent Time	Chamber O₂	Repet
5	6:40	AIR									2	9:20	0.5	
		AIR/O₂									1	8:20		
10	6:40	AIR									8	15:20	0.5	
		AIR/O₂									4	11:20		
15	6:00	AIR							1	7	30	44:40	1	
		AIR/O₂							1	4	15	27:00		
20	5:40	AIR						5	6	7	63	87:20	1.5	
		AIR/O₂						5	6	4	27	48:40		
25	5:20	AIR					5	6	8	14	119	158:00	2	
		AIR/O₂					5	6	8	7	38	75:20		
30	5:00	AIR				5	5	8	13	24	174	234:40	2.5	
		AIR/O₂				5	5	8	13	13	47	102:00		
35	4:40	AIR			3	5	9	11	18	28	244	323:20	3	
		AIR/O₂			3	5	9	11	18	15	66	142:40		
40	4:20	AIR		1	4	9	11	11	26	28	312	407:00	4	
		AIR/O₂		1	4	9	11	11	26	15	82	179:20		

250 FSW
Exceptional Exposure

Bottom Time	Time to First Stop	Gas Mix	100	90	80	70	60	50	40	30	20	Total Ascent Time	Chamber O₂	Repet
5	7:40	AIR									3	11:20	0.5	
		AIR/O₂									2	10:20		
10	7:20	AIR								2	15	25:00	0.5	
		AIR/O₂								1	8	17:00		
15	6:40	AIR							3	7	7	41	65:20	1
		AIR/O₂							3	7	4	21	42:40	
20	6:00	AIR					2	6	5	7	12	106	144:40	2
		AIR/O₂					2	6	5	7	6	35	73:00	
25	5:40	AIR				4	5	5	7	13	24	175	239:20	2.5
		AIR/O₂				4	5	5	7	13	13	47	105:40	
30	5:20	AIR			4	4	5	9	11	20	28	257	344:00	3.5
		AIR/O₂			4	4	5	9	11	20	14	70	153:20	
35	5:00	AIR	2	5	4	10	11	14	25	29	347	452:40	4	
		AIR/O₂	2	5	4	10	11	14	25	15	89	196:00		

300 FSW
Exceptional Exposure

Bottom Time	Time to First Stop	Gas Mix	100	90	80	70	60	50	40	30	20	Total Ascent Time	Chamber O₂	Repet
5	9:20	AIR									6	16:00	0.5	
		AIR/O₂									3	13:00		
10	8:20	AIR						2	5	7	32	55:00	1	
		AIR/O₂						2	5	4	16	36:20		
15	7:20	AIR				1	4	5	6	6	10	102	142:00	1.5
		AIR/O₂				1	4	5	6	6	5	35	75:20	
20	6:40	AIR	1	4	5	5	5	6	14	28	196	271:20	2.5	
		AIR/O₂	1	4	5	5	5	6	14	15	52	124:40		
25	6:40	AIR	7	4	5	5	10	12	25	29	305	409:00	3.5	
		AIR/O₂	7	4	5	5	10	12	25	15	80	180:20		

Appendix

Medication and Intravenous Flow Formulas

Medication Concentration On Hand Calculation

$$\text{concentration on hand (mg/ml)} = \frac{\text{weight on hand (mg)}}{\text{volume on hand (ml)}}$$

Volume To Be Administered

$$\text{volume to be administered (ml)} = \frac{\text{volume on hand (ml)} \times \text{desired dose (mg)}}{\text{weight on hand (mg)}}$$

Weight Based Drug Dosage

Step 1: convert patient weight to kg (pounds ÷ 2.2 = kg)

Step 2: desired dose (mg/kg)

Step 3: determine the concentration (mg ÷ ml = mg/ml)

Step 4: determine how much volume to administer: desired dose (mg) ÷ concentration (mg/ml)

Intravenous / Intraosseous Drip Rate Formula

$$\text{drops per minute (gtt/min)} = \frac{\text{total amount of fluid to be administered (ml)} \times \text{drop factor (gtt/min)}}{\text{total time in minutes}}$$

Appendix

U.S. Navy Treatment Tables – Air and Oxygen

U.S. Navy Treatment Table Indications - Oxygen Not Available
Treatment Table 1A
1. Pain relieved at less than 66 fsw.

U.S. Navy Air Table 1A		
Depth in FSW	Time in Minutes	Total Time Hrs : Min
100	30	0:30
100 to 80	20	0:50
80	12	1:02
80 to 60	20	1:22
60	30	1:52
60 to 50	10	2:02
50	30	2:32
50 to 40	10	2:42
40	30	3:12
40 to 30	10	3:22
30	60	4:22
30 to 20	10	4:32
20	60	5:32
20 to 10	10	5:42
10	120	7:42
10 to Surface	10	7:52

U.S. Navy Air Treatment Table 1A

Appendix

Air Treatment Table 1A

1. Descent rate - 20 ft/min.
2. Ascent rate - 1 ft/min.
3. Time at 100 feet includes time from the surface.

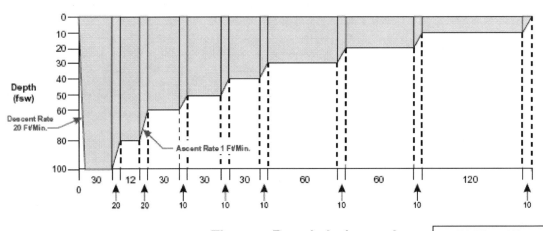

U.S. Navy Air Treatment Table 1A Graphic
US Navy Reprint from US Navy Diving Manual 6th Ed

Appendix

U.S. Navy Treatment Table Indications - Oxygen Not Available
Treatment Table 2A

1. Pain is relieved at greater than 66 fsw.

U.S. Navy Air Table 2A		
Depth in FSW	Time in Minutes	Total Time Hrs : Min
165	30	0:30
165 to 140	25	0:55
140	12	1:07
140 to 120	20	1:27
120	12	1:39
120 to 100	20	1:59
100	12	2:11
100 to 80	20	2:31
80	12	2:43
80 to 60	20	3:03
60	30	3:33
60 to 50	10	3:43
50	30	4:13
50 to 40	10	4:23
40	30	4:53
40 to 30	10	5:03
30	120	7:03
30 to 20	10	7:13
20	120	9:13
20 to 10	10	9:23
10	240	13:23
10 to Surface	10	13:33

U.S. Navy Air Treatment Table 2A

Appendix

Air Treatment Table 2A

1. Descent rate - 20 ft/min.
2. Ascent rate - 1 ft/min.
3. Time at 165 feet includes time from the surface.

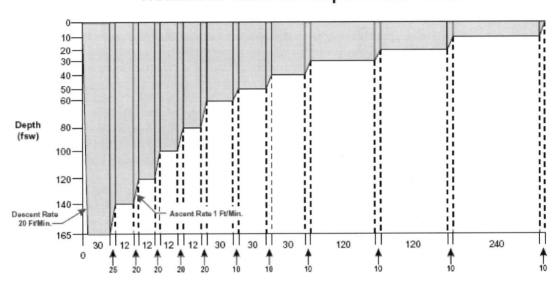

U.S. Navy Air Treatment Table 2A Graphic
US Navy Reprint from US Navy Diving Manual 6th Ed

Appendix

U.S. Navy Treatment Table Indications - Oxygen Not Available
Treatment Table 3

1. Symptoms are relieved after 30 minutes at 165 fsw.

U.S. Navy Air Table 3A		
Depth in FSW	Time in Minutes	Total Time Hrs : Min
165	30	0:30
165 to 140	25	0:55
140	12	1:07
140 to 120	20	1:27
120	12	1:39
120 to 100	20	1:59
100	12	2:11
100 to 80	20	2:31
80	12	2:43
80 to 60	20	3:03
60	30	3:33
60 to 50	10	3:43
50	30	4:13
50 to 40	10	4:23
40	30	4:53
40 to 30	10	5:03
30	720	17:03
30 to 20	10	17:13
20	120	19:13
20 to 10	10	19:23
10	120	21:23
10 to Surface	10	21:33

U.S. Navy Air Treatment Table 3

Appendix

Air Treatment Table 3

1. Descent rate - 20 ft/min.
2. Ascent rate - 1 ft/min.
3. Time at 165 feet-includes time from the surface.

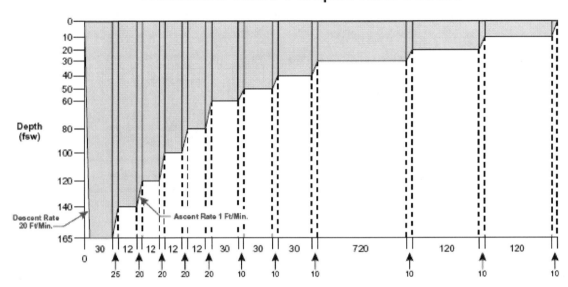

U.S. Navy Air Treatment Table 3 Graphic
US Navy Reprint from US Navy Diving Manual 6th Ed

Appendix

U.S. Navy Treatment Table Indications - Oxygen Not Available
Treatment Table 4

1. Symptoms are not relieved after 30 minutes at 165 fsw.

U.S. Navy Air Table 4		
Depth in FSW	**Time in Minutes**	**Total Time Hr : Min**
165	120	2:00
165 to 140	25	2:25
140	30	2:55
140 to 120	20	3:15
120	30	3:45
120 to 100	20	4:05
100	30	4:35
100 to 80	20	4:55
80	30	5:25
80 to 60	20	5:45
60	360	11:45
60 to 50	10	11:55
50	360	17:55
50 to 40	10	18:05
40	360	24:05
40 to 30	10	24:15
30	720	36:15
30 to 20	10	36:25
20	120	38:25
20 to 10	10	38:35
10	120	40:35
10 to Surface	1	40:36

U.S. Navy Air Treatment Table 4

Appendix

Treatment Table 4

1. Descent rate - 20 ft/min.
2. Ascent rate - 1 ft/min.
3. Time at 165 feet includes compression.
4. If only air is available, decompress on air. If oxygen is available, patient begins oxygen breathing upon arrival at 60 feet with appropriate air breaks. Both tender and patient breathe oxygen beginning 2 hours before leaving 30 feet. (see paragraph 20-5.5).
5. Ensure life-support considerations can be met before committing to a Table 4. (see paragraph 20-7.5) Internal chamber temperature should be below 85° F.
6. If oxygen breathing is interrupted, no compensatory lengthening of the table is required.
7. If switching from Treatment Table 6A or 3 at 165 feet, stay a maximum of 2 hours at 165 feet before decompressing.
8. If the chamber is equipped with a high-O_2 treatment gas, it may be administered at 165 fsw, not to exceed 3.0 ata O_2. Treatment gas is administered for 25 minutes interrupted by 5 minutes of air.

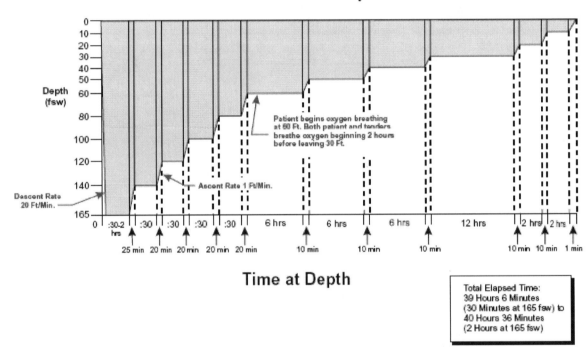

U.S. Navy Air Treatment Table 4 Graphic
US Navy Reprint from US Navy Diving Manual 6th Ed

Appendix

U.S. Navy Treatment Table Indications - Oxygen Available
Treatment Table 4
1. Worsening Type II symptoms at 60 feet.
2. Unresolved arterial gas embolism symptoms after 30 minutes at 165 feet.
3. Recurrence of symptoms 60 feet or deeper.

U.S. Navy Table 4			
Depth in FSW	Time in Minutes	Breathing Gas	Total Time Hr : Min
165	120	Mixed Gas* / Air	2:00
165 to 140	25	Mixed Gas* / Air	2:25
140	30	Mixed Gas* / Air	2:55
140 to 120	20	Mixed Gas* / Air	3:15
120	30	Mixed Gas* / Air	3:45
120 to 100	20	Mixed Gas* / Air	4:05
100	30	Mixed Gas* / Air	4:35
100 to 80	20	Mixed Gas* / Air	4:55
80	30	Mixed Gas* / Air	5:25
80 to 60	20	Mixed Gas* / Air	5:45
60	360	Oxygen	11:45
60 to 50	10	Air	11:55
50	360	Oxygen	17:55
50 to 40	10	Air	18:05
40	360	Oxygen	24:05
40 to 30	10	Air	24:15
30	720	Oxygen	36:15
30 to 20	10	Air	36:25
20	120	Oxygen	38:25
20 to 10	10	Air	38:35
10	120	Oxygen	40:35
10 to Surface	1	Oxygen	40:36
* Mixed Gas at 165 FSW to be 50/50 Heliox or 50/50 Nitrox			

U.S. Navy Oxygen Treatment Table 4

Appendix

Treatment Table 4

1. Descent rate - 20 ft/min.
2. Ascent rate - 1 ft/min.
3. Time at 165 feet includes compression.
4. If only air is available, decompress on air. If oxygen is available, patient begins oxygen breathing upon arrival at 60 feet with appropriate air breaks. Both tender and patient breathe oxygen beginning 2 hours before leaving 30 feet. (see paragraph 20-5.5).
5. Ensure life-support considerations can be met before committing to a Table 4. (see paragraph 20-7.5) Internal chamber temperature should be below 85° F.
6. If oxygen breathing is interrupted, no compensatory lengthening of the table is required.
7. If switching from Treatment Table 6A or 3 at 165 feet, stay a maximum of 2 hours at 165 feet before decompressing.
8. If the chamber is equipped with a high-O_2 treatment gas, it may be administered at 165 fsw, not to exceed 3.0 ata O_2. Treatment gas is administered for 25 minutes interrupted by 5 minutes of air.

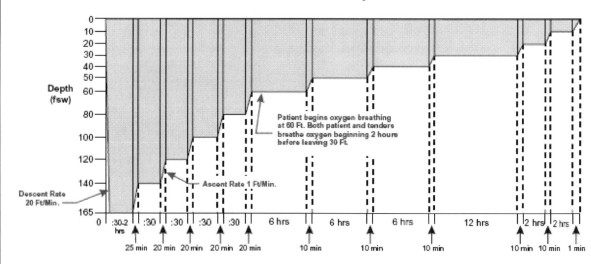

U.S. Navy Oxygen Treatment Table 4 Graphic
US Navy Reprint from US Navy Diving Manual 6th Ed

Appendix

U.S. Navy Table 4 (Modified)			
Depth in FSW	Time in Minutes	Breathing Gas	Total Time Hr : Min
165	120	Mixed Gas* / Air	2:00
165 to 140	1	Mixed Gas* / Air	2:01
140	30	Mixed Gas* / Air	2:31
140 to 120	1	Mixed Gas* / Air	2:32
120	30	Mixed Gas* / Air	3:02
120 to 100	1	Mixed Gas* / Air	3:03
100	30	Mixed Gas* / Air	3:33
100 to 80	1	Mixed Gas* / Air	3:34
80	30	Mixed Gas* / Air	4:04
80 to 60	1	Mixed Gas* / Air	4:05
60	20	Oxygen	4:25
60	5	Air	4:30
60	20	Oxygen	4:50
60	5	Air	4:55
60	20	Oxygen	5:15
60	5	Air	5:20
60 to 30	30	Oxygen	5:50
30	15	Air	6:05
30	60	Oxygen	7:05
30	15	Air	7:20
30	60	Oxygen	8:20
30 to Surface	30	Oxygen	8:50
* Mixed Gas at 165 FSW to be 50/50 Heliox or 50/50 Nitrox			

Table 6-1 - U.S. Navy Oxygen Treatment Table 4 Modified

Appendix

Treatment Table 5

1. Type I symptoms relieved within 10 minutes of arrival at 60 feet with normal pre-treatment neuro examination.
2. Asymptomatic missed decompression.
3. Treated and resolved in-water symptoms.
4. Exceeded Sur-D surface interval, asymptomatic.

U.S. Navy Table 5			
Depth in FSW	Time in Minutes	Breathing Gas	Total Time Hr : Min
60	20	Oxygen	0:20
60	5	Air	0:25
60	20	Oxygen	0:45
60 to 30	30	Oxygen	1:15
30	5	Air	1:20
30	20	Oxygen	1:40
30	5	Air	1:45
30 to Surface	30	Oxygen	2:15

U.S. Navy Oxygen Treatment Table 5

Appendix

Treatment Table 5

1. Descent rate - 20 ft/min.
2. Ascent rate - Not to exceed 1 ft/min. Do not compensate for slower ascent rates. Compensate for faster rates by halting the ascent.
3. Time on oxygen begins on arrival at 60 feet.
4. If oxygen breathing must be interrupted because of CNS Oxygen Toxicity, allow 15 minutes after the reaction has entirely subsided and resume schedule at point of interruption (see paragraph 20-7.11.1.1)
5. Treatment Table may be extended two oxygen-breathing periods at the 30-foot stop. No air break required between oxygen-breathing periods or prior to ascent.
6. Tender breathes 100 percent O_2 during ascent from the 30-foot stop to the surface. If the tender had a previous hyperbaric exposure in the previous 18 hours, an additional 20 minutes of oxygen breathing is required prior to ascent.

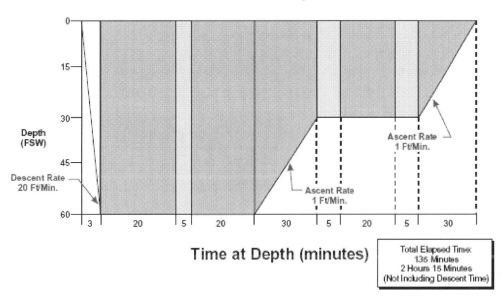

U.S. Navy Oxygen Treatment Table 5 Graphic
US Navy Reprint from US Navy Diving Manual 6th Ed

Appendix

U.S. Navy Table 5 With Extension at 60 fsw			
Depth in FSW	Time in Minutes	Breathing Gas	Total Time Hr : Min
60	20	Oxygen	0:20
60	5	Air	0:25
60	20	Oxygen	0:45
60	5	Air	0:50
60	20	Oxygen	1:10
60	5	Air	1:15
60 to 30	30	Oxygen	1:45
30	5	Air	1:50
30	20	Oxygen	2:10
30	5	Air	2:15
30 to Surface	30	Oxygen	2:45

U.S. Navy Oxygen Treatment Table 5 with Extension @ 60 fsw

U.S. Navy Table 5 With Extension at 60 fsw and at 30 fsw			
Depth in FSW	Time in Minutes	Breathing Gas	Total Time Hr : Min
60	20	Oxygen	0:20
60	5	Air	0:25
60	20	Oxygen	0:45
60	5	Air	0:50
60	20	Oxygen	1:10
60	5	Air	1:15
60 to 30	30	Oxygen	1:45
30	5	Air	1:50
30	20	Oxygen	2:10
30	5	Air	2:15
30	20	Oxygen	2:35
30	5	Air	2:40
30 to Surface	30	Oxygen	3:10

U.S. Navy Oxygen Treatment Table 5 with Extensions @ 60 fsw & 30 fsw

Appendix

Treatment Table 6
1. Type I symptoms not resolved within 10 minutes at 60 feet or where neuro examination not done.
2. Recurrence of symptoms shallower than 60 feet.
3. Type II or arterial gas embolism symptoms responding to an initial 60-foot recompression.
4. Type II symptoms after diving less 100 feet and presenting within 6-8 hour post.

U.S. Navy Table 6			
Depth in FSW	Time in Minutes	Breathing Gas	Total Time Hr : Min
60	20	Oxygen	0:20
60	5	Air	0:25
60	20	Oxygen	0:45
60	5	Air	0:50
60	20	Oxygen	1:10
60	5	Air	1:15
60 to 30	30	Oxygen	1:45
30	15	Air	2:00
30	60	Oxygen	3:00
30	15	Air	3:15
30	60	Oxygen	4:15
30 to Surface	30	Oxygen	4:45

U.S. Navy Oxygen Treatment Table 6

Appendix

Treatment Table 6

1. Descent rate - 20 ft/min.
2. Ascent rate - Not to exceed 1 ft/min. Do not compensate for slower ascent rates. Compensate for faster rates by halting the ascent.
3. Time on oxygen begins on arrival at 60 feet.
4. If oxygen breathing must be interrupted because of CNS Oxygen Toxicity, allow 15 minutes after the reaction has entirely subsided and resume schedule at point of interruption (see paragraph 20-7.11.1.1).
5. Table 6 can be lengthened up to 2 additional 25-minute periods at 60 feet (20 minutes on oxygen and 5 minutes on air), or up to 2 additional 75-minute periods at 30 feet (15 minutes on air and 60 minutes on oxygen), or both.
6. Tender breathes 100 percent O_2 during the last 30 min. at 30 fsw and during ascent to the surface for an unmodified table or where there has been only a single extension at 30 or 60 feet. If there has been more than one extension, the O_2 breathing at 30 feet is increased to 60 minutes. If the tender had a hyperbaric exposure within the past 18 hours an additional 60-minute O_2 period is taken at 30 feet.

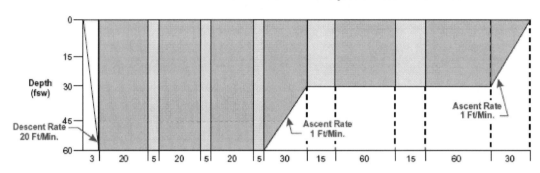

U.S. Navy Oxygen Treatment Table 6 Graphic
US Navy Reprint from US Navy Diving Manual 6th Ed

Appendix

U.S. Navy Table 6 With Extension at 60 fsw			
Depth in FSW	Time in Minutes	Breathing Gas	Total Time Hr : Min
60	20	Oxygen	0:20
60	5	Air	0:25
60	20	Oxygen	0:45
60	5	Air	0:50
60	20	Oxygen	1:10
60	5	Air	1:15
60	20	Oxygen	1:35
60	5	Air	1:40
60 to 30	30	Oxygen	2:10
30	15	Air	2:25
30	60	Oxygen	3:25
30	15	Air	3:40
30	60	Oxygen	4:40
30 to Surface	30	Oxygen	5:10

U.S. Navy Oxygen Treatment Table 6 with Extension @ 60 fsw

U.S. Navy Table 6 With Extension at 60 fsw and 30 fsw			
Depth in FSW	Time in Minutes	Breathing Gas	Total Time Hr : Min
60	20	Oxygen	0:20
60	5	Air	0:25
60	20	Oxygen	0:45
60	5	Air	0:50
60	20	Oxygen	1:10
60	5	Air	1:15
60	20	Oxygen	1:35
60	5	Air	1:40
60 to 30	30	Oxygen	2:10
30	15	Air	2:25
30	60	Oxygen	3:25
30	15	Air	3:40
30	60	Oxygen	4:40
30	15	Air	4:55
30	60	Oxygen	5:55
30 to Surface	30	Oxygen	6:25

U.S. Navy Oxygen Treatment Table 6 with Extensions @ 60 fsw & 30 fsw

Appendix

Treatment Table 6A

1. Arterial gas embolism not responding at 60 feet but resolving within 30 minutes at 165 feet where initially 20 minutes or less is spent at 60 feet.
2. Symptomatic blow-up from greater than 60 feet.

U.S. Navy Table 6A			
Depth in FSW	Time in Minutes	Breathing Gas	Total Time Hr : Min
165	25	Mixed *	0:25
165	5	Air	0:30
165 to 60	35	Mixed *	1:05
60	20	Oxygen	1:25
60	5	Air	1:30
60	20	Oxygen	1:50
60	5	Air	1:55
60	20	Oxygen	2:15
60	5	Air	2:20
60 to 30	30	Oxygen	2:50
30	15	Air	3:05
30	60	Oxygen	4:05
30	15	Air	4:20
30	60	Oxygen	5:20
30 to Surface	30	Oxygen	5:50
* Mixed Gas at 165 FSW to be 50/50 Heliox or 50/50 Nitrox			

U.S. Navy Oxygen / Mixed Gas Treatment Table 6A

Appendix

Treatment Table 6A

1. Descent rate - 20 ft/min.
2. Ascent rate - 165 fsw to 60 fsw not to exceed 3 ft/min, 60 fsw and shallower, not to exceed 1 ft/min. Do not compensate for slower ascent rates. Compensate for faster rates by halting the ascent.
3. Time at treatment depth does not include compression time.
4. Table begins with initial compression to depth of 60 fsw. If initial treatment was at 60 feet, up to 20 minutes may be spent at 60 feet before compression to 165 fsw. Contact a Diving Medical Officer.
5. If a chamber is equipped with a high-O_2 treatment gas, it may be administered at 165 fsw and shallower, not to exceed 3.0 ata O_2 in accordance with paragraph 20-7.10. Treatment gas is administered for 25 minutes interrupted by 5 minutes of air. Treatment gas is breathed during ascent from the treatment depth to 60 fsw.
6. Deeper than 60 feet, if treatment gas must be interrupted because of CNS oxygen toxicity, allow 15 minutes after the reaction has entirely subsided before resuming treatment gas. The time off treatment gas is counted as part of the time at treatment depth. If at 60 feet or shallower and oxygen breathing must be interrupted because of CNS oxygen toxicity, allow 15 minutes after the reaction has entirely subsided and resume schedule at point of interruption (see paragraph 20-7.11.1.1).
7. Table 6A can be lengthened up to 2 additional 25-minute periods at 60 feet (20 minutes on oxygen and 5 minutes on air), or up to 2 additional 75-minute periods at 30 feet (60 minutes on oxygen and 15 minutes on air), or both.
8. Tender breathes 100 percent O_2 during the last 60 minutes at 30 fsw and during ascent to the surface for an unmodified table or where there has been only a single extension at 30 or 60 fsw. If there has been more than one extension, the O_2 breathing at 30 fsw is increased to 90 minutes. If the tender had a hyperbaric exposure within the past 18 hours, an additional 60 minute O_2 breathing period is taken at 30 fsw.
9. If significant improvement is not obtained within 30 minutes at 165 feet, consult with a Diving Medical Officer before switching to Treatment Table 4.

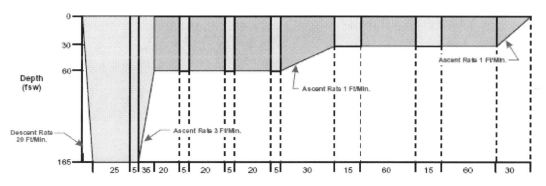

U.S. Navy Oxygen / Mixed Gas Treatment Table 6A Graphic
US Navy Reprint from US Navy Diving Manual 6th Ed

Appendix

Treatment Table 7

1. Type II or arterial gas embolism symptoms needing more time at 60 feet.
2. Arterial gas embolism symptoms relieved within 30 minutes at 165 feet but where more than 20 minutes spent at 60 feet during initial recompression.

U.S. Navy Table 7			
Depth in FSW	Time in Hours	Breathing Gas	Total Time Hr : Min
60	12 Hrs Minimum	Oxygen 20 / 5 Air	12:00
58 to 40	6 Hrs	Oxygen 20 / 5 Air	18:00
40 to 20	10 Hrs	Oxygen 20 / 5 Air	28:00
20 to 4	16 Hrs	Oxygen 20 / 5 Air	44:00
4	4 Hrs	Oxygen 20 / 5 Air	52:00
4 to Surface	4 Minutes	Oxygen	52:04

U.S. Navy Oxygen Treatment Table 7

Appendix

Treatment Table 7

1. Table begins upon arrival at 60 feet. Arrival at 60 feet is accomplished by initial treatment on Table 6, 6A or 4. If initial treatment has progressed to a depth shallower than 60 feet, compress to 60 feet at 20 ft/min to begin Table 7.
2. Maximum duration at 60 feet is unlimited. Remain at 60 feet a minimum of 12 hours unless overriding circumstances dictate earlier decompression.
3. Patient begins oxygen breathing periods at 60 feet. Tender need breathe only chamber atmosphere throughout. If oxygen breathing is interrupted, no lengthening of the table is required.
4. Minimum chamber O_2 concentration is 19 percent. Maximum CO_2 concentration is 1.5 percent SEV (11.4 mmHg). Maximum chamber internal temperature is 85°F (paragraph 20-7.5).
5. Decompression starts with a 2-foot upward excursion from 60 to 58 feet. Decompress with stops every 2 feet for times shown in profile below. Ascent time between stops is approximately 30 seconds. Stop time begins with ascent from deeper to next shallower step. Stop at 4 feet for 4 hours and then ascend to the surface at 1 ft/min.
6. Ensure chamber life-support requirements can be met before committing to a Treatment Table 7.
7. A Diving Medical Officer should be consulted before committing to this treatment table.

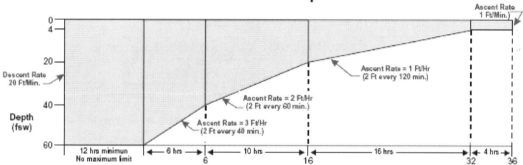

U.S. Navy Oxygen Treatment Table 7 Graphic
US Navy Reprint from US Navy Diving Manual 6th Ed

Appendix

Treatment Table 8

1. Deep blowup from surface supplied helium-oxygen dives.

	U.S. Navy Table 8		
Depth in FSW	Maximum Time In Hours	Breathing Gas	2 – FSW Stop Times in Minutes
225	0.5	Mixed Gas *	5
165	3	Mixed Gas **	12
140	5	Mixed Gas **	15
120	8	Mixed Gas **	20
100	11	Mixed Gas **	25
80	15	Mixed Gas **	30
60	Unlimited Time	Oxygen ***	40
40	Unlimited Time	Oxygen ***	60
20	Unlimited Time	Oxygen ***	120

Treatment Table 8

1. Enter the table at the depth which is exactly equal to or next greater than the deepest depth attained in the recompression. The descent rate is as fast as tolerable.

2. The maximum time that can be spent at the deepest depth is shown in the second column. The maximum time for 225 fsw is 30 minutes; for 165 fsw, 3 hours. For an asymptomatic diver, the maximum time at depth is 30 minutes for depths exceeding 165 fsw and 2 hours for depths equal to or shallower than 165 fsw.

3. Decompression is begun with a 2-fsw reduction in pressure if the depth is an even number. Decompression is begun with a 3-fsw reduction in pressure if the depth is an odd number. Subsequent stops are carried out every 2 fsw. Stop times are given in column three. The stop time begins when leaving the previous depth. Ascend to the next stop in approximately 30 seconds.

4. Stop times apply to all stops within the band up to the next quoted depth. For example, for ascent from 165 fsw, stops for 12 minutes are made at 162 fsw and at every two-foot interval to 140 fsw. At 140 fsw, the stop time becomes 15 minutes. When traveling from 225 fsw, the 166-foot stop is 5 minutes; the 164-foot stop is 12 minutes. Once begun, decompression is continuous. For example, when decompressing from 225 feet, ascent is not halted at 165 fsw for 3 hours. However, ascent may be halted at 60 fsw and shallower for any desired period of time.

5. While deeper than 165 fsw, a helium-oxygen mixture with 16-36 percent oxygen may be breathed by mask to reduce narcosis. A 64/36 helium-oxygen mixture is the preferred treatment gas. At 165 fsw and shallower, a HeO_2 or N_2O_2 mix with a ppO_2 not to exceed 3.0 ata may be given to the diver as a treatment gas. At 60 fsw and shallower, pure oxygen may be given to the divers as a treatment gas. For all treatment gases (HeO_2, N_2O_2 and O_2), a schedule of 25 minutes on gas and 5 minutes on chamber air should be followed for a total of four cycles. Additional oxygen may be given at 60 fsw after a 2-hour interval of chamber air. See Treatment Table 7 for guidance. If high O_2 breathing is interrupted, no lengthening of the table is required.

6. To avoid loss of the chamber seal, ascent may be halted at 4 fsw and the total remaining stop time of 240 minutes taken at this depth. Ascend directly to the surface upon completion of the required time.

7. Total ascent time from 225 fsw is 56 hours, 29 minutes. For a 165-fsw recompression, total ascent time is 53 hours, 52 minutes, and for a 60-fsw recompression, 36 hours, 0 minutes.

Depth (fsw)	Max Time at Initial Treatment Depth (hours)	2-fsw Stop Times (minutes)
225	0.5	5
165	3	12
140	5	15
120	8	20
100	11	25
80	15	30
60	Unlimited	40
40	Unlimited	60
20	Unlimited	120

U.S. Navy Oxygen Treatment Table 8 Graphic
US Navy Reprint from US Navy Diving Manual 6th Ed

Appendix

Treatment Table 9
1. Residual symptoms remaining after initial treatment of AGE/DCS.
2. Selected cases of carbon monoxide or cyanide poisoning.
3. Smoke inhalation.

U.S. Navy 9			
Depth in FSW	Time in Minutes	Breathing Gas	Total Time Hr : Min : Sec
45	30	Oxygen	0:30:00
45	5	Air	0:35:00
45	30	Oxygen	1:05:00
45	5	Air	1:10:00
45	30	Oxygen	1:40:00
45 to Surface	2:15	Oxygen	1:42:15

U.S. Navy Oxygen Treatment Table 9

Appendix

Alternative Oxygen Treatment Tables

COMEX Table Cx 30

1. Arterial gas embolism not responding at initial 60 feet on USN TT6A but shows improvement at 100 feet.
2. Type II symptoms not responding to an initial USN TT6.
3. Type II symptoms after diving to greater than 100 feet.

Comex Table 30			
Depth in FSW	Time in Minutes	Breathing Gas	Total Time Hrs : Min
100	25	Mixed Gas *	0:25
100	5	Air	0:30
100	25	Mixed Gas *	0:55
100	5	Air	1:00
100 to 80	5	Air	1:05
100 to 80	25	Mixed Gas *	1:30
80	5	Air	1:35
80	25	Mixed Gas *	2:00
80 to 60	5	Air	2:05
80 to 60	25	Mixed Gas *	2:30
60	20	Oxygen	2:50
60	5	Air	2:55
60	20	Oxygen	3:15
60	5	Air	3:20
60	20	Oxygen	3:40
60	5	Air	3:45
60 to 30	30	Oxygen	4:15
30	15	Air	4:30
30	60	Oxygen	5:30
30	15	Air	5:45
30	60	Oxygen	6:45
30 to Surface	30	Oxygen	7:15
* Mixed Gas to be 50/50 Heliox or 50/50 Nitrox			

COMEX 30 Oxygen / Mixed Gas Treatment Table

Appendix

Royal Navy Table 71 & 72
1. Patient in poor condition requiring greater depth than 165 feet.
2. Patient in poor condition after 2 hours at 165 needing slow decompression.

Royal Navy Table 71			
Depth in FSW	Stops / Ascents Hrs : Min	Breathing Gas	Rate of Ascent FSW / Hour
230	0:30	Mixed Gas *	Hold
230 to 208	0:07	Mixed Gas *	198
208 to 168	2:00	Mixed Gas *	20
168 to 129	4:00	Mixed Gas *	10
129 to 96	5:00	Mixed Gas *	6
96 to 66	6:00	Mixed Gas *	5
66 to 33	10:00	Oxygen **	3
33 to Surface	20:00	Oxygen **	1.6
Royal Navy Table 72			
165	2:00	Mixed Gas *	Hold
164 to 129	3:40	Mixed Gas *	10
Complete with Royal Navy Table 71 at Depth of 129 FSW			
* Mixed Gas to be of Helium/Oxygen or Nitrogen/Oxygen NOT TO EXCEED 3.0 ATA O_2			
** Oxygen Periods to be 20 Minutes Followed by 5 Minutes Air			

Royal Navy Oxygen / Mixed Gas Treatment Tables 71 & 72

Appendix

Lambertsen/SOSI Table 7A
1. Patient shows symptoms under pressure.
2. Patient requires recompression deeper than 165 feet.
3. Patient requires extended decompression.

\multicolumn{5}{c}{Lambertsen Table 7A}				
Depth in FSW	Ascent Rate	Chamber Atmosphere **	Breathing Gas	Total Time Hrs : Min
Final Treatment Depth *	1 fsw per 4 min.	Air or Heliox	Chamber Atmosphere	30 minutes plus ascent to 165 fsw
165 to 150	1 fsw per 4 min.	Air	Air	1:00
150 to 100	1 fsw per 6 min.	Air	Air	5:00
100 to 70	1 fsw per 10 min.	Air	50/50 Nitrox or Heliox Available; 5 cycles of 30 minutes mixed gas, 30 minutes air.	5:00
70 to 60	1 fsw per 15 min.	Air	Air	2:30
60 to 40	1 fsw per 15 min.	Air	5 cycles of 30 minutes of oxygen, 30 minutes air.	5:00
40 to 30	1 fsw per 15 min.	Air	Air	2:30
30 to 20	1 fsw per 30 min.	Air	5 cycles of 30 minutes of oxygen, 30 minutes air. (Includes Tender)	5:00
20 to 10	1 fsw per 30 min.	Air	Air	5:00
10 to 2	1 fsw per 30 min.	Air	4 cycles of 30 minutes of oxygen, 30 minutes air	4:00
2 to Surface	1 fsw per 30 min.	Air	Oxygen	1:00

* Final Treatment Depth: On AIR Limited to 200 fsw, ascend to 165 after 30 minute HOLD in 1 minute.
On Heliox go to depth of relief plus 33 fsw (No deeper than dive) Hold for 30 minutes and then ascend to 165 fsw at a rate of 1 fsw per 4 minutes.

Lambertsen Treatment Table 7A

Appendix

Cornerstone Treatment Table

1. Type II symptoms after diving greater than 100 feet with long delay in presenting. (1 to 7 days)

\multicolumn{4}{c}{Cornerstone Table}			
Depth in FSW	Time in Minutes	Breathing Gas	Total Time Hrs : Min
165	25	50/50 Nitrox**	0:25
165	5	Air	0:30
165*	25	50/50 Nitrox	0:55
165*	5	Air	1:00
165 to 140	10	50/50 Nitrox	1:10
140	10	50/50 Nitrox	1:20
140 to 120	10	50/50 Nitrox	1:30
120	5	Air	1:35
120	10	50/50 Nitrox***	1:45
120 to 100	10	50/50 Nitrox	1:55
100	5	Air	2:00
100	15	50/50 Nitrox	2:15
100 to 80	10	50/50 Nitrox	2:25
80	5	Air	2:30
80	15	50/50 Nitrox	2:45
80 to 60	10	50/50 Nitrox	2:55
60	5	Air	3:00
Complete Treatment on USN Table 6	285	Oxygen	7:45

* Optional Extension at 165 fsw
** Helium / Oxygen Treatment Mix May Be Substituted
***40 He or N / 60 O_2 Concentration May Be Used from 120 to 60 fsw if Available.

Cornerstone Oxygen / Mixed Gas Deep Treatment Table

Appendix

Conversion Factors

The following are useful and necessary conversion factors and data for the diver medic.

Temperature Conversion from Fahrenheit to Celsius and Celsius to Fahrenheit.

Formula: °F to °C: °C = (°F − 32) ÷ 1.8

°C to °F: °F = (1.8 x °C) + 32

Temperature Conversions

Temperature Conversions				
Celsius	Fahrenheit	Kelvin	Rankine	Newton
300.00	572.00	573.15	1031.67	99.00
290.00	554.00	563.15	1013.67	95.70
280.00	536.00	553.15	995.67	92.40
270.00	518.00	543.15	977.67	89.10
260.00	500.00	533.15	959.67	85.80
250.00	482.00	523.15	941.67	82.50
240.00	464.00	513.15	923.67	79.20
230.00	446.00	503.15	905.67	75.90
220.00	428.00	493.15	887.67	72.60
210.00	410.00	483.15	869.67	69.30
200.00	392.00	473.15	851.67	66.00
190.00	374.00	463.15	833.67	62.70
180.00	356.00	453.15	815.67	59.40
170.00	338.00	443.15	797.67	56.10
160.00	320.00	433.15	779.67	52.80
150.00	302.00	423.15	761.67	49.50
140.00	284.00	413.15	743.67	46.20
130.00	266.00	403.15	725.67	42.90
120.00	248.00	393.15	707.67	39.60

Appendix

Celsius	Fahrenheit	Kelvin	Rankine	Newton
110.00	230.00	383.15	689.67	36.30
100.00	212.00	373.15	671.67	33.00
90.00	194.00	363.15	653.67	29.70
80.00	176.00	353.15	635.67	26.40
70.00	158.00	343.15	617.67	23.10
60.00	140.00	333.15	599.67	19.80
50.00	122.00	323.15	581.67	16.50
40.00	104.00	313.15	563.67	13.20
30.00	86.00	303.15	545.67	9.90
20.00	68.00	293.15	527.67	6.60
10.00	50.00	283.15	509.67	3.30
0.00	32.00	273.15	491.67	0.00
−10.00	14.00	263.15	473.67	−3.30
−20.00	−4.00	253.15	455.67	−6.60
−30.00	−22.00	243.15	437.67	−9.90
−40.00	−40.00	233.15	419.67	−13.20
−50.00	−58.00	223.15	401.67	−16.50
−60.00	−76.00	213.15	383.67	−19.80
−70.00	−94.00	203.15	365.67	−23.10
−80.00	−112.00	193.15	347.67	−26.40
−90.00	−130.00	183.15	329.67	−29.70
−100.00	−148.00	173.15	311.67	−33.00
−110.00	−166.00	163.15	293.67	−36.30
−120.00	−184.00	153.15	275.67	−39.60
−130.00	−202.00	143.15	257.67	−42.90
−140.00	−220.00	133.15	239.67	−46.20
−150.00	−238.00	123.15	221.67	−49.50
−160.00	−256.00	113.15	203.67	−52.80

Appendix

Celsius	Fahrenheit	Kelvin	Rankine	Newton
−170.00	−274.00	103.15	185.67	−56.10
−180.00	−292.00	93.15	167.67	−59.40
−190.00	−310.00	83.15	149.67	−62.70
−200.00	−328.00	73.15	131.67	−66.00
−210.00	−346.00	63.15	113.67	−69.30
−220.00	−364.00	53.15	95.67	−72.60
−230.00	−382.00	43.15	77.67	−75.90
−240.00	−400.00	33.15	59.67	−79.20
−250.00	−418.00	23.15	41.67	−82.50
−260.00	−436.00	13.15	23.67	−85.80
−273.15	−459.67	0.00	0.00	−90.14

Pressure (Hydrostatic) Conversions

Hydrostatic Pressure Conversions					
	ATA Atmospheres Absolute	FSW Feet Sea Water	MSW Meters Sea Water	PSI Pounds Square Inch	kPa Kilopascals
1 ATA =	1	33	10	14.7	101.325
1 FSW =	0.030	1	0.3048	0.445	3.063
1 MSW =	0.099	3.28	1	1.45	10.0
1 PSI =	0.068	2.25	0.68	1	6.8965
1 kPa =	0.009869	0.326	0.1	0.145	1

Appendix

Pressure (Barometric) Conversions

Barometric Pressure Conversions					
	ATM Atmosphere	Bars	mmHg Millimeters Mercury	In Hg Inches Mercury	PSI Pounds Square Inch
1 ATM =	1	1.013	760	29.92	14.7
1 Bar =	.9869	1	750.1	29.53	14.51
1 mmHg =	.00316	.001333	1	.03937	.01934
1 In Hg =	.0334	.03386	25.4	1	.4910
1 PSI =	.06804	.06895	51.70	2.035	1

Volume Conversions

Volume Conversions					
	Ft^3 Cubic Foot	Lt Liter	Gal Gallon	M^3 Cubic Meter	
1 Ft^3 =	1	28.32	7.48	0.028	
1 Liter =	0.035	1	0.264	0.001	
1 Gallon =	0.13	3.79	1	0.0038	
1 M^3 =	35.31	1000	264.2	1	

Length Conversions

Common Metric / Imperial Length Conversions								
	Inch	Foot	Yard	Mile (Statue)	Millimeter	Centimeter	Meter	Kilometer
1 Inch =	1	.08333	.0278	.0000158	25.40	2.540	.02540	.0000254
1 Foot =	12	1	.333	.0001893	304.8	30.48	.3048	.0003048
1 Yard =	36	3	1	.0005682	914.4036	91.44036	.9144036	.000914404
1 Mile =	63,360	5280	1760	1	1,609,344	160,934.4	1,609.34	1.60934
1 Millimeter =	.03937	.003281	.0.1094	25.4	1	.1	.001	.000001
1 Centimeter=	.3937	.032808	.01094	.00000621	10	1	.01	.00001
1 Meter =	39.37	3.2808	1.0936	.0006214	1,000	100	1	.001
1 Kilometer =	39370.1	3280.84	1093.6	.6214	1,000,000	100,000	1000	1

Appendix

Perimeter Formulas

Perimeter Formulas	
Square	4 * side
Rectangle	2 * (length + width)
Parallelogram	2 * (side1 + side2)
Triangle	side1 + side2 + side3
Regular n-polygon	n * side
Trapezoid	height * (base1 + base2) / 2
Trapezoid	base1 + base2 + height * [csc(theta1) + csc(theta2)]
Circle	2 * pi * radius

Area Formulas

Area Formulas	
Square	$side^2$
Rectangle	length * width
Parallelogram	base * height
Triangle	base * height / 2
Regular n-polygon	(1/4) * n * $side^2$ * cot(pi/n)
Trapezoid	height * (base1 + base2) / 2
Circle	pi * $radius^2$
Ellipse	pi * radius1 * radius2
Cube (surface)	6 * $side^2$
Sphere (surface)	4 * pi * $radius^2$
Cylinder (surface of side)	perimeter of circle * height 2 * pi * radius * height
Cylinder (whole surface)	Areas of top and bottom circles + Area of the side 2 (pi * $radius^2$) + 2 * pi * radius * height
Cone (surface)	pi * radius * side
Torus (surface)	pi^2 * ($radius2^2$ - $radius1^2$)

Appendix

Volume Formulas

Volume Formulas	
Cube	$side^3$
Rectangular Prism	side1 * side2 * side3
Sphere	$(4/3) * pi * radius^3$
Ellipsoid	(4/3) * pi * radius1 * radius2 * radius3
Cylinder	$pi * radius^2 * height$
Cone	$(1/3) * pi * radius^2 * height$
Pyramid	(1/3) * (base area) * height
Torus	$(1/4) * pi^2 * (r1 + r2) * (r1 - r2)^2$

Section Answer Keys
Section 1 – History of Diving and Hyperbarics

Mix and Match

1. c
2. f
3. e
4. b
5. a
6. d
7. m
8. o
9. l
10. h
11. i
12. n
13. k
14. j
15. g

Review Questions

1. d
2. c
3. d
4. a
5. b
6. c
7. a
8. c
9. a
10. a
11. c
12. c
13. b
14. d
15. a
16. d
17. a

Section 2 – Roles and Responsibilities of the Diver Medic

Review Questions

1. a
2. a
3. a
4. a
5. c
6. a
7. a
8. d
9. a

Answer Keys

Section 3 - Diving Physics

Mix and Match

1. f
2. e
3. n
4. b
5. g
6. h
7. a
8. c
9. d
10. l
11. m
12. o
13. i
14. j
15. k

Review Questions

1. a
2. a
3. b
4. c
5. a
6. a
7. b
8. c
9. b
10. a
11. d
12. a
13. b
14. a
15. a
16. a
17. b
18. a
19. c
20. b
21. a
22. a
23. d
24. a
25. a

Gas Consumption Review

1. b
2. a
3. b

Answer Keys

Section 4 – Anatomy and Physiology

Fill In the Blanks

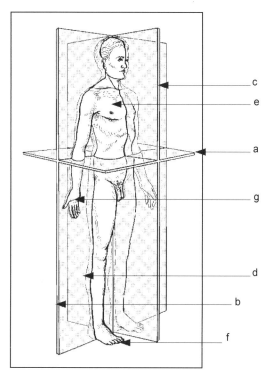

Label Directional Views

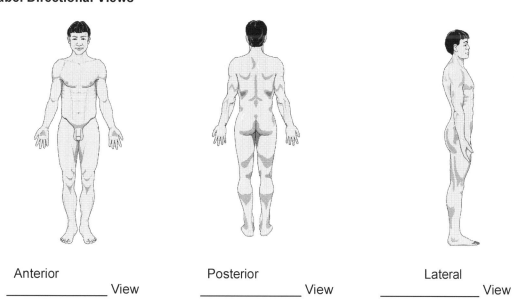

Anterior
_____ View

Posterior
_____ View

Lateral
_____ View

Answer Keys

Labeling Exercise

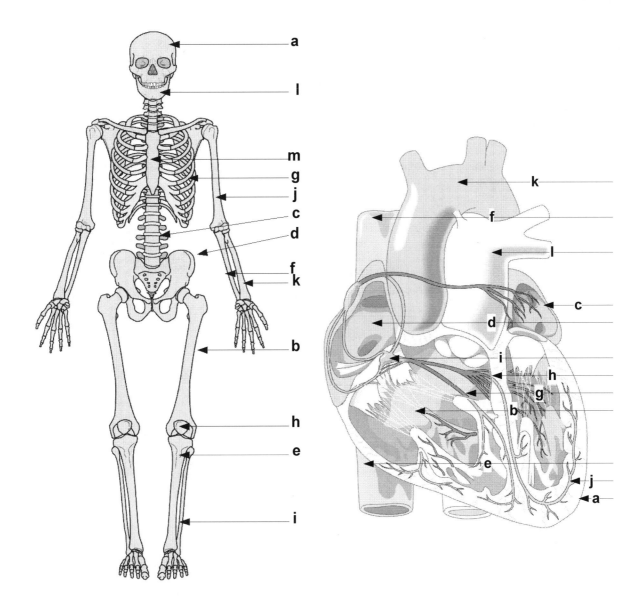

Cardiac / Vascular Review Questions

1. c
2. d
3. d
4. b
5. c
6. d
7. a
8. a
9. b
10. b
11. d
12. a
13. a
14. b
15. a

Answer Keys

Respiratory System Review

Labeling Exercise

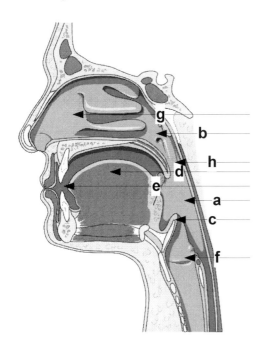
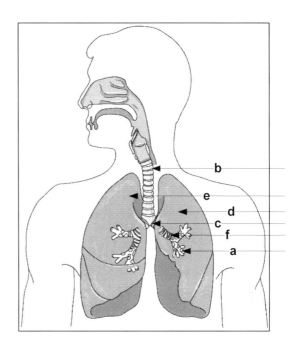

Respiratory Review Questions

1. c
2. c
3. a
4. d
5. c
6. c
7. b
8. a
9. b

Answer Keys

Nervous System Review

Labeling Exercise

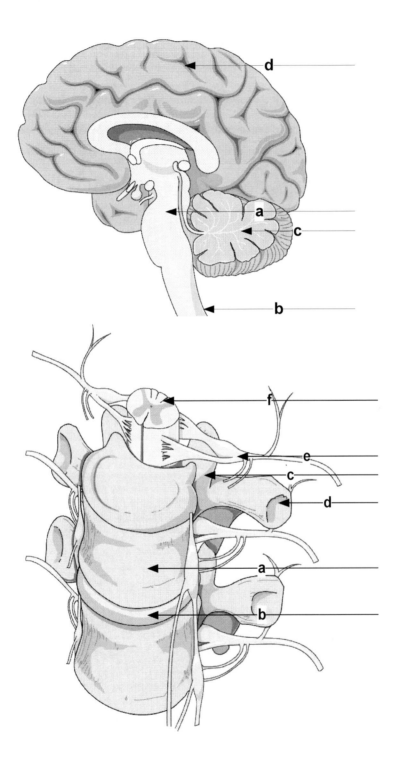

Answer Keys

Section 5 - Patient Assessment

Matching
1. i
2. a
3. h
4. g
5. j
6. l
7. k
8. b
9. c
10. e
11. d
12. f

Matching Sample
1. c
2. a
3. e
4. f
5. d
6. b

Matching OPQRST
1. b
2. e
3. a
4. f
5. c
6. d

Matching DCAP-BTLS
1. b
2. e
3. f
4. d
5. g
6. h
7. a
8. c

Patient Assessment Review Questions
1. d
2. a
3. a
4. a
5. b
6. c
7. b
8. b
9. a
10. d
11. b
12. c
13. c
14. d
15. b
16. a
17. a
18. a
19. a
20. d

Neurologic Assessment Review Questions
1. a
2. a
3. b
4. d
5. a
6. c
7. a
8. a
9. a
10. d

Answer Keys

Section 6 - The Tables – Decompression and Recompression

Diving Tables Review Questions
1. c
2. c
3. a
4. b
5. b
6. a
7. a
8. a
9. c
10. b
11. a
12. c
13. a
14. c
15. c

Treatment Tables Review Questions
1. b
2. a
3. c
4. a
5. a
6. a
7. a.
8. b
9. d
10. a
11. a
12. d
13. a
14. b
15. b

Section 7 - Hyperbaric Chambers

Hyperbaric Chamber Review Questions
1. a
2. a
3. d
4. d
5. a
6. d
7. a
8. a
9. a
10. b
11. d
12. a
13. c
14. a
15. a
16. a
17. a
18. c
19. b
20. c
21. b
22. a
23. b
24. c
25. a
26. b
27. a
28. d
29. d
30. a
31. a
32. a

Answer Keys

Section 8 - Pressure Injuries and Illness

Fill In the Blanks

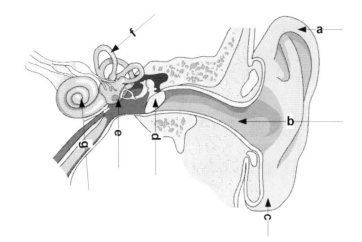

Pressure Injuries and Illness Review Questions

1. a
2. d
3. d
4. c
5. a
6. c
7. c
8. d
9. c
10. b
11. c
12. b
13. a
14. d
15. a
16. c
17. a
18. d
19. d
20. d
21. a
22. a
23. b
24. a
25. a
26. a
27. d
28. d
29. d
30. d
31. a
32. b
33. b
34. a
35. b
36. a
37. a
38. a
39. a
40. d
41. d
42. b
43. b
44. a
45. a

Answer Keys

Section 9 - Medical and Marine Injuries

Medical Review Questions

1. a	15. c
2. c	16. b
3. a	17. a
4. d	18. a
5. a	19. d
6. d	20. a
7. a	21. c
8. a	22. a
9. a	23. a
10. a	24. d
11. d	25. a
12. a	26. c
13. a	27. c
14. a	28. a

Section 10 - Airway and Breathing

Airway & Breathing Review Questions

1. a	14. d	27. a
2. b	15. d	28. a
3. b	16. d	29. c
4. c	17. c	30. a
5. c	18. b	31. c
6. c	19. a	32. c
7. a	20. a	33. a
8. c	21. c	34. c
9. a	22. c	35. b
10. a	23. a	36. b
11. c	24. a	37. d
12. d	25. b	38. a
13. a	26. a	40. c
		41. b

Answer Keys

Section 10 - Continued

Identify the Airways

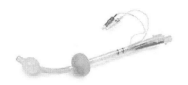

a. ETC CombiTube

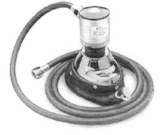

b. Flow Restricted Demand Ventilator

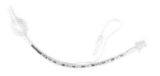

c. Endotracheal Tube

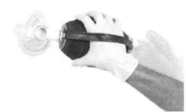

d. Bag Valve Mask

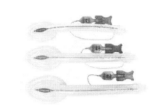

e. Laryngeal Mask Airways

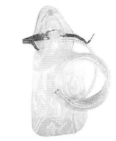

f. Non-Rebreather O2 Mask

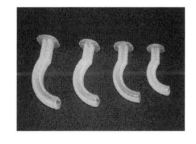

g. Oropharyngeal Airways

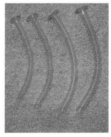
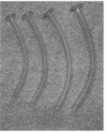

h. Nasopharyngeal Airways

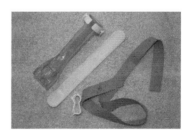

i. S.A.L.T. Airway

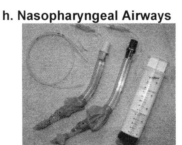

j. KING Airways

Answer Keys

Section 10 - Continued

Fill in the Blanks

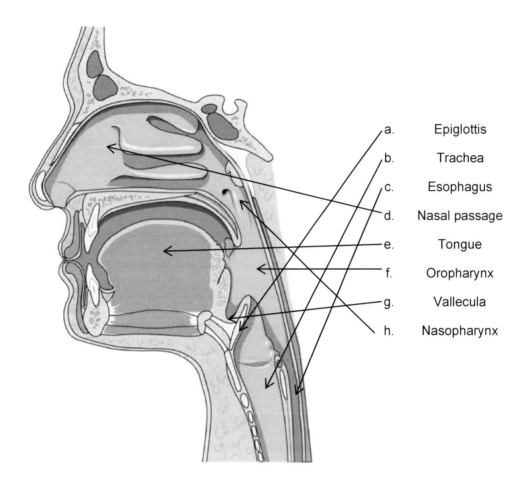

a. Epiglottis
b. Trachea
c. Esophagus
d. Nasal passage
e. Tongue
f. Oropharynx
g. Vallecula
h. Nasopharynx

Answer Keys

Section 11 - Vascular Access and Medication Administration

Fill in the Blanks

Six Patient Rights
1. Right Patient
2. Right Medication
3. Right Dose
4. Right Route
5. Right Time
6. Right Documentation

1. 20 mg
2. 1 mg
3. 1 mg

1. 1.25 ml
2. 4 ml

1. 75 gtt/min
2. 125 gtt/min
3. 25 gtt/min

Mix and Match

Percutaneous Route: d, e

Enteral Route: g

Parenteral Route: a, b, c, f

Medication Concentration On Hand Calculation

Volume To Be Administered Calculation

Intravenous / Intraosseous Drip Rate Calculation

Review Questions
1. a
2. d
3. a
4. a
5. d
6. c
7. c
8. a
9. d
10. d
11. b
12. d
13. a
14. d
15. a
16. b
17. a
18. d
19. b
20. b
21. c
22. a
23. a
24. b
25. a

Mix and Match

1. b
2. f
3. a
4. g
5. h
6. i
7. e
8. j
9. c
10. d

Answer Keys

Section 12 - Soft Tissue Injury

Fill in the Blanks

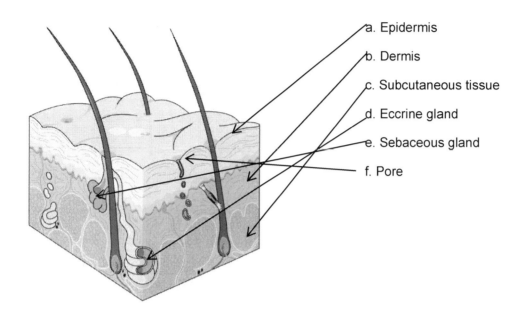

a. Epidermis
b. Dermis
c. Subcutaneous tissue
d. Eccrine gland
e. Sebaceous gland
f. Pore

Mix and Match

1. f
2. g
3. e
4. a
5. h
6. i
7. j
8. c
9. d
10. b

Soft Tissue Review Questions

1. b
2. a
3. b
4. a
5. b
6. a
7. d
8. a
9. c
10. a
11. c
12. d
13. d
14. c
15. c
16. b
17. b
18. a
19. c
20. a
21. d
22. a
23. d
24. c
25. a
26. a
27. a
28. b
29. d
30. a

Answer Keys

Labeling Exercise – Rule of Nines

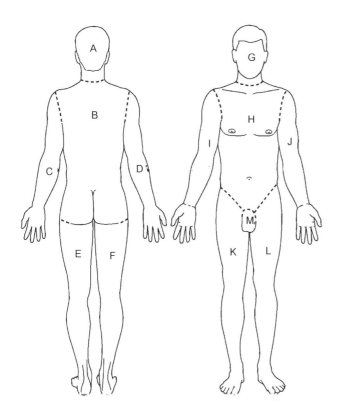

A. 4.5 %
B. 18 %
C. 4.5 %
D. 4.5 %
E. 9 %
F. 9 %
G. 4.5 %
H. 18 %
I. 4.5 %
J. 4.5 %
K. 9 %
L. 9 %
M. 1 %

Answer Keys

Section 13 – Musculoskeletal Injury

Fill in the Blanks

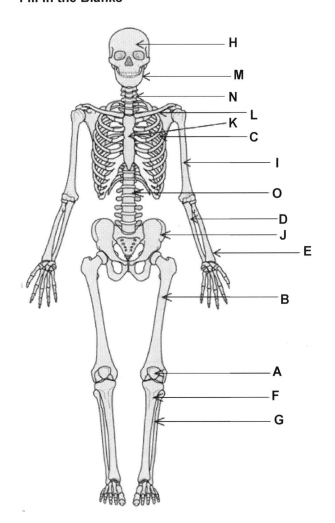

A. Patella
B. Femur
C. Ribs
D. Ulna
E. Radius
F. Tibia
G. Fibula
H. Skull
I. Humerus
J. Pelvis
K. Sternum
L. Clavicle
M. Mandible
N. Cervical vertebrae
O. Lumbar vertebrae

Mix and Match

1. d
2. a
3. f
4. b
5. j
6. h
7. i
8. e
9. g
10. c

Labeling Exercise

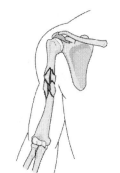

A. Comminuted

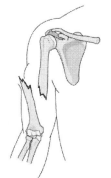

B. Open / Compound / Angulated

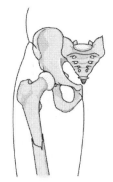

C. Spiral

Answer Keys

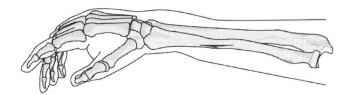
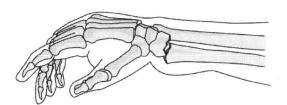

D. Greenstick E. Closed / Angulation

Musculoskeletal Review Questions

1. c	7. a	14. a
2. a	8. b	15. b
3. b	9. a	16. a
4. c	10. d	17. b
5. b	11. b	18. c
6. a	12. c	19. d
	13. d	20. d

Section 14 – Cardiac Emergencies

Mix and Match
1. c
2. j
3. e
4. g
5. h
6. d
7. a
8. f
9. b
10. i

Cardiac Review Questions
1. a
2. c
3. a
4. b
5. c
6. c
7. a
8. b
9. a
10. b
11. a
12. b
13. a
14. a
15. c

Answer Keys

Section 15 – Related Medical Procedures

Procedures Review Questions

1. b	7. b	14. a
2. d	8. c	15. c
3. a	9. b	16. a
4. c	10. b	17. a
5. d	11. d	18. c
6. a	12. b / d	19. a
	13. a	20. c

Section 16 – Saturation Diving Issues

Saturation Review Questions

1. a	6. a	11. a
2. b	7. c	12. d
3. a	8. b	13. a
4. b	9. b	14. b
5. a	10. a	15. a

Section 17 – Live Bait

Review Questions

1. b	11. a	21. a
2. d	12. b	22. b
3. b	13. b	23. b
4. b	14. a	24. b
5. a	15. a	25. b
6. a	16. d	26. b
7. b	17. b	27. a
8. b	18. a	28. b
9. a	19. c	29. c
10. c	20. a	30. a

Made in United States
Troutdale, OR
09/21/2024

23024929R00093